» Praise for Myatt Murphy «

"It has always been a pleasure to work with Myatt. I consider him one of the top writers in the fitness industry and congratulate him on yet another top-notch publication."

—JUAN CARLOS "JC" SANTANA,
director of the Institute of Human Performance in Boca Raton, Florida

"I have worked with Myatt for many years, and I've never met anyone who is more current on all aspects of the fitness industry. He has an incredible ability to discern fact from fad. If Myatt wrote it, it's worth reading!"

—STEVE LISCHIN, BS, MS, NASM,
celebrity trainer and head of Steve Lischin Fitness in Manhattan

"Over the years, I have worked with many people in the publishing industry, as well as the fitness industry. Myatt Murphy is one of the rare individuals who truly has an understanding of the strength and fitness world. He's not just a writer, he's a writer with knowledge and passion for his topics. Myatt is a true professional in every sense of the word and continues to turn out the highest quality information available."

—C. J. MURPHY, MFS, SSC, CFT,
multiple award-winning trainer and head instructor
of Total Performance Sports in Everett, Massachusetts

"Myatt is a "fact sleuth" for exercisers, searching out the best available information and crafting it into readable and entertaining material. You can trust his work to help you accomplish all of your fitness goals."

—DIXIE STANFORTH, MS,
Department of Kinesiology and Health Education
at the University of Texas in Austin, Texas

"Murphy raises the bar yet again with *Men's Health's Ultimate Dumbbell Guide*. If progress and performance are as important to you as they are to me, you need look no further than the insight and in-depth understanding of fitness and performance that he adds to each and every book he puts his pen to. No hype. No hidden agenda. *Men's Health's Ultimate Dumbbell Guide* is just about getting results."

—JOHN MACLAREN, BS, CPT,
former US Navy SEAL, celebrity and performance athlete trainer

"Myatt understands the nuances of motivating people to strive to get healthier and be more fit. He continues to get the message of fitness out to the public, writing innovative, realistic, and imaginative books and articles. With an uncanny insight into what people want to know about their health and well-being, Myatt has a passion and dedication for providing thoughtful and useful information in his articles and books. He's simply one of the best in the business."

—HEATHER DILLINGER,
certification specialist for the Aerobic and Fitness Association of America

Men'sHealth

ULTIMATE
DUMBBELL
GUIDE

Men'sHealth

ULTIMATE
DUMBBELL
GUIDE

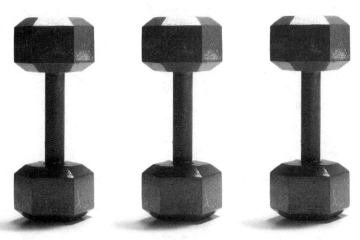

**MORE THAN 21,000 MOVES DESIGNED TO BUILD
MUSCLE, INCREASE STRENGTH, AND BURN FAT**

MYATT MURPHY

RODALE

The information in this book is meant to supplement, not replace, proper exercise training. All forms of exercise pose some inherent risks. The editors and publisher advise readers to take full responsibility for their safety and know their limits. Before practicing the exercises in this book, be sure that your equipment is well maintained, and do not take risks beyond your level of experience, aptitude, training, and fitness. The exercise and dietary programs in this book are not intended as a substitute for any exercise routine or dietary regimen that may have been prescribed by your doctor. As with all exercise and dietary programs, you should get your doctor's approval before beginning.

Mention of specific companies, organizations, or authorities in this book does not imply endorsement by the author or publisher, nor does mention of specific companies, organizations, or authorities imply that they endorse this book, its author, or the publisher.

Internet addresses and telephone numbers given in this book were accurate at the time it went to press.

Rodale books may be purchased for business or promotional use or for special sales. For information, please write to:
Special Markets Department, Rodale Inc., 733 Third Avenue, New York, NY 10017

Men's Health® is a registered trademark of Rodale Inc.

Printed in the United States of America
Rodale Inc. makes every effort to use acid-free ♾, recycled paper ♻.

BOOK DESIGN BY SUSAN P. EUGSTER
PHOTOGRAPHS BY MITCH MANDEL / RODALE IMAGES

Library of Congress Cataloging-in-Publication Data

Murphy, Myatt.
    Men's Health ultimate dumbbell guide : more than 21,000 moves designed to build muscle, increase strength, and burn fat / Myatt Murphy.
        p.   cm.
    Includes index.
    ISBN-13 978-1-60529-635-7 hardcover
    ISBN-10 1-60529-635-X hardcover
    ISBN-13 978-1-59486-487-2 paperback
    ISBN-10 1-59486-487-X paperback
    1. Dumbbells.   2. Physical fitness for men.   3. Exercise for men.   I. Men's Health Books.
II. Title.
    GV547.4.M87   2007
    613.7'0449—dc22
                                                                                    2007010647

Distributed to the trade by Macmillan

2   4   6   8   10   9   7   5   3   1   hardcover
          6   8   10   9   7   5   paperback

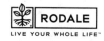

We inspire and enable people to improve their lives and the world around them

For more of our products visit **rodalestore.com** or call 800-848-4735

TO MY DAD,

whose exercise advice changed my life
and guided me on the path of doing the same
for millions of men and women worldwide.
If this book gets you into great shape,
he's the one to thank.

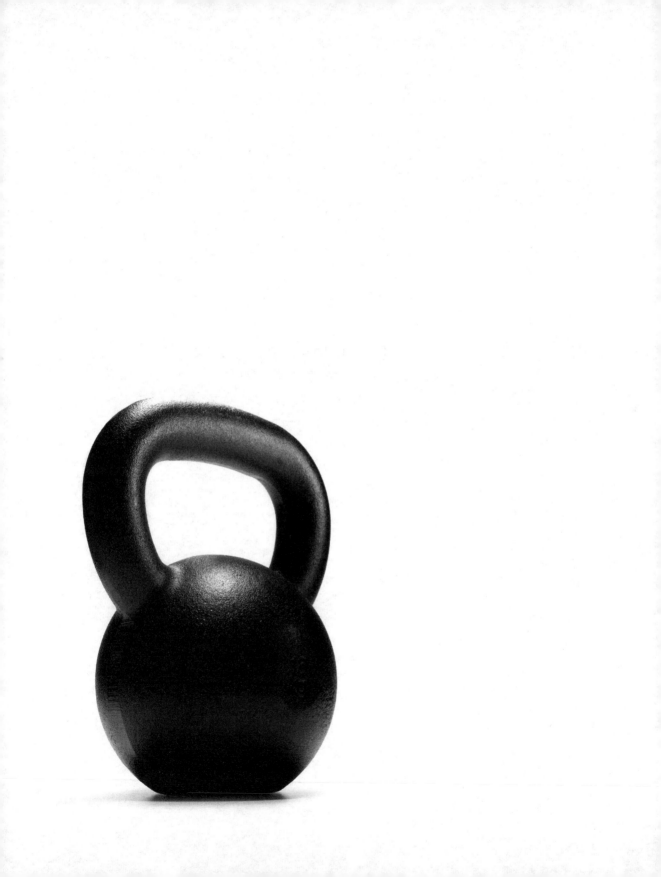

Contents

Acknowledgments

I WANT TO THANK every editor who has—in one way or another—allowed me to deliver my take on exercise and fitness with millions of readers worldwide for 14 years now. I've been blessed to write more than 620 features for 50-plus international magazines and work with some of the best writers and editors in the business—and have been inspired by a variety of successful book authors whose work taught me to write books that readers can use not just today, but for a lifetime. Hopefully, I haven't left anyone off this list of professionals that I admire—but here goes: Rochelle Udell, Lucy Danziger, Gabrielle Studenmund, Stephen George, Malcolm Gladwell, Bobby Lee, Mike Carlson, Nora Ephron, Pamela Miller, Michael Losier, Jennifer Fields, Laura Gilbert, Jerome Groopman, Jeff Csatari, Stephenie Meyer, Rosie Amodio, Jim Karas, Duane Swierczynski, Ed Dwyer, Elizabeth O'Brian, Jennifer Walters, Trevor Thieme, Nicole Dorsey, Jeffrey Gitomer, Albert Baime, Alex Strauss, Beth Bischoff, Gordon Bass, Emily Spilko, Rhonda Byrne, Denise Brodey, Frederic Delavier, Stephanie Young, Meaghan Buchan, Gunnar Waldman, Scott Quill, Phillip Rhodes, Stephen Perrine, Nichele Hoskins, Mary Christ, Su Reid, Gail O'Connor, Abigail Walch, Dana Points, Lisa Delany, Tamar Geller, David Kalmansohn, Timothy Ferriss, Jerry Kindela, Nina Willdorf, and Alison Ashton.

I've also had the opportunity to know hundreds of personal trainers, exercise physiologists, nutritionists, and sports psychologists, with whom I've either studied under, interviewed, trained with and/or ghostwritten for: Joy Bauer, Harley Pasternak, Ian K. Smith, Judith S. Beck, Jillian Michaels, Tosca Reno, Brenda Watson, Barbara Rolls, Marion Nestle, John Berardi, Melissa Perlman, Nicholas DiNubile, William J. Kraemer, David Pearson, Ellington Darden, Minna Lessig, Mark Hyman, Kurt Brungardt, Brad Schoenfeld, Wayne Westcott, Michael Thurmond, Bob Cooley, Brooke Siler, Pamela Peeke, Robin McKenzie, and Eric Harr, to name just a few. It's been a pleasure to work with nearly every top fitness professional in the business, and as I say in each and every book I write—there's no greater education than that.

I also want to thank everyone at Rodale who gave me the chance to show you that dumbbells truly have infinite possibilities: David Zinczenko, Zachary Schisgal, Courtney Conroy, Mitch Mandel, Susan Eugster, Nancy Bailey, Keith Biery, Amy Kovalski, Troy Schneider, Jessica Settle, Erik Nelson, Adrienne Bearden, Mark Sirinsky, and everyone else who worked on this project. I'm sure that there are probably a lot of behind-the-scenes people that I'm unaware of—because a lot of hands take over after it leaves my desk—and if that's you, thank you very much.

Finally, thanks, Dad. I've said it in other books and I'll say it forever—thank you for teaching me about exercise when I was young. If you hadn't shared everything that you knew about fitness with me, I never would have been able to share everything I know about fitness with the readers in this book.

Myatt Murphy

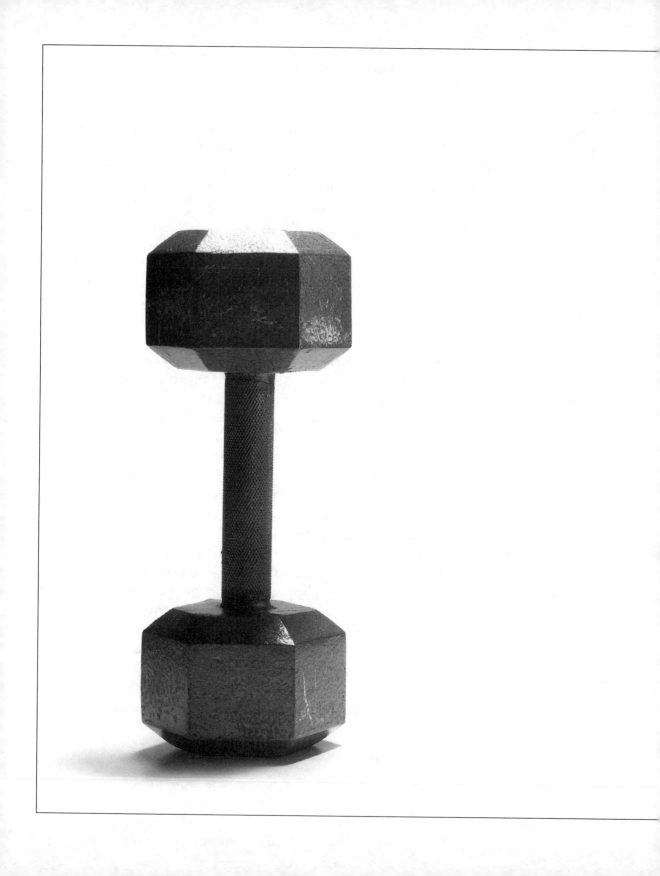

PART ONE

THE TRUTH ABOUT DUMBBELLS

One

TWO WEIGHTS ... MANY OPTIONS!

"THERE ARE LITERALLY HUNDREDS of exercises you can do with dumbbells!"

Does that phrase sound familiar? It should. Whether you are new to exercise or have been doing it for longer than your body would care to remember, you've probably heard at least one exercise expert—if not hundreds—make that exact point when it comes to the benefits of this incredibly versatile exercise tool: the dumbbell.

Well, I have something to reveal to you.

They're all wrong.

That's right. Every single expert, every single personal trainer, every single coach, and every single exercise physiologist you've ever heard go on record as saying there are literally *hundreds* of exercises you can do with dumbbells wasn't exactly being honest with you. That's because there aren't *hundreds* of exercises you can do with dumbbells.

There are exactly 4,988 exercises.

And I should know because every single one of them is in this book.

That's right. If you've bought this book, you have a decision to make when it comes to exercise. To be more accurate, you actually have 4,988 decisions to make. Because if you've ever been perplexed by what to do with that old pair of dumbbells you bought a long time ago—but haven't been using lately—this book will show you more ways to challenge your muscles than you'd honestly ever need in your lifetime.

So why are all those "exercise experts" confused about how many options are available to you? Who knows. Perhaps many of them don't realize themselves how many exercises a pair of dumbbells can yield. Or perhaps they lack the know-how to devise that many interesting muscle-building moves. Or maybe it's simply because they just wouldn't even know where to begin trying to explain each and every variation that's possible. Either that or their publisher told them they had no interest in printing a 2,000-page, 20-pound book—even though it doesn't require all that space if you organize them as I have in this book. Regardless of their reasons, that's why this specific book about dumbbells gives you an edge where others simply fail.

THE MASTER MOVES

The secret to this book is in its order. You'll learn how to perform a series of 130 basic dumbbell exercises, or what I call Master Moves. These particular exercises are some of the best basic exercises you can do with a pair of dumbbells. If you've ever trained with dumbbells, you'll recognize some of them, while others may be more advanced than you're used to.

After that, you'll learn just how easy it is to add a variation to any of the Master Moves to create hundreds and, ultimately, thousands of "new" exercises that are either more effective, more challenging, or most important, more interesting to your muscles. From that point forward, you'll never look at a single pair of dumbbells again without thinking about how limitless their uses are. Finally, I'll show you ways to take those thousands of moves and easily organize them into exercise routines that match your personal fitness goals—no matter what they are.

GO BEYOND THE 4,988

Are there really 4,988 exercises you can do with dumbbells? I have to come clean and tell you that 4,988 is actually incorrect. That's because 4,988 would be an understatement. All of the exercises in this book can be done either with no additional equipment save a set of dumbbells or by using a few ordinary exercise equipment accessories like a weight bench or a Swiss ball, for example. If I added other less-common exercise equipment into the mix (such as cable pulleys, resistance cords, etc.), I could have shown you even more. But instead of making you spend more money, this book lets you do even more than 4,988 exercises by doing what no other exercise book has ever done before—showing you how to make your own.

Before I explain, let me ask you to do something first. Place a set of dumbbells down by the outsides of your feet—if you don't have a pair in front of you, just go through the motions with an imaginary pair. (This is the only exercise in this book that's strictly for your brain.) Now, bend down, grab a dumbbell in each hand, and stand back up—palms facing in. Curl them both up to your shoulders, rest the ends of the dumbbells on the front of your shoulders, then squat down. Stand back up, then press the weights over your head. Twist to the left, twist to the right, then lower the weights back down to your shoulders. Curl them back down until your arms are straight, then place them back on the floor.

Congratulations! Technically you've just worked almost every major muscle group in your body simultaneously—including your legs, back, butt, shoulders, triceps, biceps, and core muscles—using what I call the "Murphy Multilift." Actually, that move had no name until just now. By definition, it's really nothing more than a Deadlift/ Hammer Curl/Front Squat/Shoulder Press/ Standing Oblique Twist, because those are the five exercises I combined into one move.

The point? Many of the unique exercises you've read about in magazines or seen on TV are nothing more than exercises you'll find in this book—merged together into one multistep exercise. That's why, in addition to the thousands of moves I'm about to show you, I'm going to reveal just how easy it is to combine dumbbell exercises to create new and interesting ones all your own. The result creates:

- Exercises tailor-made to match your specific exercise goals.

- Exercises that can be as long or as short as you need them to be.

- Exercises that hit all of the muscles you need to train in one time-saving shot.

And lest I forget, exercises you can name after yourself. Why not? After all, you created it, didn't you?

Now let's get started!

Two

WHY YOU NEED DUMBBELLS

BEFORE I SHOW YOU the thousands of possible exercises you can do with dumbbells, it's important to know the eight main reasons why they're one of the most important pieces of exercise equipment you could ever use.

You see, maybe you bought a pair of dumbbells because they were convenient or inexpensive, compared to a pricey gym membership or those multipurposed home-gym contraptions they sell on late-night television for 60 easy payments of "insert your latest paycheck here____." But most people have no idea how much of an impact dumbbells actually make when it comes to how well your body can potentially transform as a result of exercise. In fact, the cheapest item on the block may very well be the most effective when it comes to your overall fitness.

DUMBBELLS GIVE YOU THE MOST VERSATILITY

Now I'm sure you're thinking, "All right already. Dumbbells are the only pieces of exercise equipment I'll ever need. I get it!" But it bears repeating because unlike most exercise-specific machines you may see in gyms, which can cost upward of $500 to $10,000 and yet allow you to do only as little as *one* single exercise on them, an ordinary pair of dumbbells offers you thousands.

Even the dumbbell's closest counterpart—the barbell—can't offer as many options because most barbell exercises require you to use both hands to handle the weight, which severely limits how many single-handed, seated, Swiss ball, and other creative exercises you can do with them. When you do the math, one pair of dumbbells costs you pennies per exercise, once you know all the exercises they offer, of course.

DUMBBELLS KEEP YOUR MUSCLES GUESSING AND GROWING

Because of all that versatility, your best bet for seeing consistent results from exercise—for life—starts with investing in dumbbells.

■ ■ ■

Do you remember the first time you ever did something that required your undivided attention—like the day you couldn't wait to learn how to drive, for example? Do you also remember how difficult it was when you first got behind the wheel? Every part of your body felt like it was on edge as you tried to focus on everything—your driving, your surroundings, the road, etc.—all at once!

After a while, the excitement of driving suddenly disappeared, didn't it? After doing it over and over again, it suddenly became easier and easier to do without your ever realizing it. You probably drive so instinctively now that you barely devote one-tenth as much attention to it as you did on that very first day. That is exactly how your muscles react when they are given the same exercises to do every single workout.

Exercise physiologists, strength coaches, and other exercise experts all agree that your muscles adapt to an exercise quickly—usually within performing the exercise four to six times. After that, they get bored and quickly learn how to do that exercise using less effort, less energy, and fewer muscle fibers. The unfortunate outcome: You stop seeing results, no matter how long you keep exercising—weeks, months, even years. That's the reason why most people hit a peak where, all of a sudden, their bodies stop improving like they once did when they first started an exercise program.

Even the slightest change to an exercise can make a huge difference that reminds your muscles to pay attention. Most home exercise machines allow you to do anywhere from 12 to 50 different exercises, but unfortunately, once you're through with those, there's really no room left to grow. The versatility of dumbbells, however, allows you to switch any overdone exercise with hundreds of other similar options that constantly challenge your muscles. With thousands to choose from, it's virtually impossible for your muscles to get bored.

DUMBBELLS LEAVE YOU MORE ELBOW ROOM

Unless you plan on investing in a wide assortment of dumbbells of all weights and sizes, these mini muscle builders generally take up far less space in your house than your average home gym. If even that sounds too cumbersome, you can also opt for a pair of adjustable dumbbells that let you add or remove weight plates to create whatever load you need.

There are also more space-friendly models—called *selectorized adjustable dumbbells*—that can reduce the amount of space an entire set of dumbbells normally takes up. These types of dumbbells keep all of the weight plates in one convenient spot—usually on a sturdy rack—with each plate resting inside the other like a stack of cups. These fancier models let you add as much or as little weight as you need with just a change of a pin, a turn of a dial, or a press of a button (depending on which type of selectorized dumbbell set you buy). I'll explain the differences among all three styles in Chapter Three, but regardless of which type works best for you, all three are great bets if you like your home exercise convenient when you're doing it—and out of plain sight when you're not.

DUMBBELLS GIVE YOUR ARMS THEIR INDEPENDENCE

Most of the exercise machines you'll find in gyms and health clubs require you to use both hands to push or pull a weight this way or that way. Even a barbell still requires you to use both hands for nearly every exercise you can do with it. But how often do you ask your arms to perform the same task at the same time? Maybe that's the case when you pick up a box, for example, but there are virtually millions of daily tasks—grabbing a suitcase, throwing a ball, holding a child, pulling on a stuck door, etc.—that have you using one arm instead of two. That's what makes dumbbells ideal for strengthening your body in the same way that you use it all day long.

Lifting dumbbells allows you to do what experts call "unilateral" training. In layman's terms, it's when you train one limb (an arm or a leg) at a time. Not only does this allow you to train your muscles in the way you typically use them throughout the day, but it also helps make up for any imbalances you may already have. You see, most people have one arm—and one leg—that's stronger than the other. That may not mean much to you, but it means a world of difference to your body. That's because your muscles develop and grow to their fullest potential *only* when they're pushed beyond the stresses that they're used to.

Using machines and barbells—which force you to use both arms at the same time—can rob your weaker arm of results by having your stronger arm do more of the work when you exercise. Conversely, your stronger arm can also get cheated out of results, especially if your weaker arm tires out first as you exercise. Because machine and barbell exercises require you to use both hands, your stronger arm never gets pushed hard enough to evoke as many muscle-building changes, leaving it less developed than it could be. This effect doesn't just pertain to arm exercises but all upper-body exercises because you need your arms to train your back, chest, and shoulders. Dumbbells allow each arm to work independently—when one arm gets too tired, the other can usually keep going, depending on the exercise.

DUMBBELLS IMPROVE YOUR OVERALL BALANCE

Sitting nice and comfortably in a gym exercise machine may help you focus on nothing but the muscles you're looking to train when you use it, but it doesn't teach those same muscles to work with the rest of your body the way working out with dumbbells does. Yet another advantage to using a pair of dumbbells to pull off the same exercises instead.

Throughout the day, your body keeps itself balanced by recruiting additional mini-stabilizing muscles—otherwise known as your proprioceptive muscles. These are the little neurological helpers that instinctively react to your movements 24-7, making tiny adjustments to your posture continuously to keep your body in perfect alignment and in balance.

Working out with dumbbells—especially when you work one arm or one leg at a time—overloads your proprioceptive muscles as they try to keep your body stable during many commonly unstable exercises. This leaves them working just as hard as the muscles you're trying to reshape and rebuild, improving your sense of balance and coordination naturally as a side benefit.

This "extra effort" your body has to exert using dumbbells is the main reason why you can never seem to lift as much weight using two dumbbells as you can when using a barbell or a machine. But don't worry, because it doesn't matter how much weight you lift to exhaust your muscles; the point is to exhaust them so they respond in turn by improving themselves—either by getting stronger, bigger, leaner, etc. Dumbbells are equally effective at accomplishing that goal, with better balance being another perk that indirectly comes along for the ride.

DUMBBELLS OFFER A SAFER WORKOUT

Some people believe that dumbbells are the most unsafe piece of equipment for lifting, and that expensive gym machines and barbells are easier to handle and can be grabbed at a moment's notice by a spotter. However, the truth is dumbbells can be far safer for you for several reasons.

As I mentioned, while you can't use as much weight when using dumbbells compared to doing the same exercise on a machine or with a barbell, your body still sees the same muscle-building results. From a safety standpoint, not having to use as much weight to exhaust your muscles means less wear and tear on your body, especially for your joints and your spine.

Machines and barbells also limit your body's range of motion by forcing you to push or pull along a specific pathway. For example, if you sat down at a machine, grabbed a pair of handles by your shoulders, and pressed them upward, your muscles would have to move the weight in the exact direction the handles require you to move them. Sit down and grab a barbell and you have a little bit more flexibility to adjust yourself by either moving your arms an inch or two either backward or forward as you press the weight up. However, your hands still stay spaced the same distance from each other as you press and lower the barbell.

The problem with limiting your range of motion is that it causes your muscles and joints to work the same way over and over again. This can make them more susceptible to repetitive-use injuries—nagging chronic issues caused by overusing certain parts of your body, especially the joints, for an extended period of time. Additionally, the angle of these kinds of exercises may not be one where your body works its best.

With dumbbells, you are able to adjust each arm individually, letting you bring the weights forward or backward and closer in or farther apart. This allows you to naturally align your arms as you raise and lower the weight. It also slightly changes where they are positioned each and every time you lift them, minimizing the amount of wear and tear on your joints.

Finally, dumbbells let you push your muscles to the limit without worrying if there's a spotter around to rescue you from a barbell that's too heavy for you. Doing shoulder presses, bench presses, squats, and the other exercises you'll find in this book using a barbell can be tricky, especially if you find yourself too tired to complete a repetition. But with dumbbells, there are no bars to get trapped under. So long as you have a floor that can handle the shock, it's easy enough to drop the weights if you find yourself too exhausted to control the weights properly.

DUMBBELLS WORK— NO MATTER WHAT YOUR SIZE

As fancy as many gym exercise machines may be, most of them—as I just mentioned—force you to work within a specific range of motion. However, many of them also force you to grab handles or lie down and adjust footpads and backrests that may or may not be the right width for your body type.

What many people don't know is that most machines are built to accommodate the average-size person. But if you're either above or below average height, your arms or legs are longer or shorter than average, or your shoulders are wider or more narrow than average, you're at a biomechanical disadvantage when you work out on any machine that doesn't accommodate you. If you've ever used a machine that "just didn't feel as comfortable as it should have," odds

are your range of motion was restricted because of your body type.

Even though most machines have adjustable seats, arm pads, and lever arms that aim to make them more comfortable to use, there are still limits to their range, and some may not fit the very small or very large person. With dumbbells, your size doesn't matter because they allow you to work within your own natural range of motion with every single exercise.

DUMBBELLS GIVE YOU AN ATHLETIC EDGE

For all the reasons already discussed—better balance, more muscle development, fewer injuries—it should be obvious why training with dumbbells can naturally improve your sports performance—or your performance during almost any real-life activity you may find yourself doing where you may be seeking improvement.

Dumbbells can take your performance to another level by allowing you to perform exercises that condition the muscle groups you use to make specific movements you often use in your sport. Dumbbells are versatile enough to use while mimicking movements like golf swings, for example, whereas trying to perform the same action with a barbell or exercise machine could prove very difficult. For a stronger swing on the golf course or in the batting cages, picking up a dumbbell and performing the same swing can train the *exact* muscles you use specifically for that motion. Need more stability moving side-to-side on the tennis or basketball courts? Grabbing a pair of dumbbells and lunging across the floor the way you typically travel on the court strengthens the *exact* muscles that you use when performing that same motion when playing your sport. In other words, with the thousands of options available for you to try, it's easy to find the right exercises for mimicking the movements where you need more strength and/or stability. You'll gain a powerful edge over your competition.

Three

HOW TO PICK THE PERFECT SET TO MATCH YOUR MUSCLES

YOU'RE READING A BOOK that offers you thousands of exercises you can do with dumbbells. But no matter how much useful information is inside it, it's worthless to your body if you don't have access to these valuable pieces of equipment in the first place. The right set of dumbbells for you depends on your exercise experience, goals, and preferences.

If you're a newcomer to weight training, your best choice would be a set that allows you to get results but doesn't require a huge investment. However, if you've been weight training for a while and getting stronger each and every week, investing in dumbbells capable of fulfilling your needs as you get stronger and require more weight is a wise decision.

If you lack even the smallest amount of space to store several sets of dumbbells, opting for an adjustable pair that allows you to add or remove weight to create several pairs in one may be a smart buy. However, if you hate having to change weight plates constantly and want to be able to grab any size dumbbell you may need in an instant—and have the room to house them—purchasing an entire rack of dumbbells that range in weight may be your solution.

Everyone's preferences are different. But I can tell you that although it's possible to do every exercise in this book with a light pair of dumbbells, it's not enough to have only one pair. In order to get your muscles to respond to exercise, you have to place them under the right amount of stress. For some muscles—and certain exercises—being able to achieve that may only take a pair of dumbbells that weigh 5 pounds each. For other muscles—and other exercises—that may take a pair that weighs 10 pounds, or 20, or 30, or 40, etc. So investing in a few different sizes of dumbbells can prevent you from ever having to use a weight that's not heavy enough to make your muscles respond or one that's not light enough to allow you to do the exercise safely and effectively.

There are three styles of dumbbells you can choose from to get started. Depending on how much you're willing to spend, how much room you have, and how patient you are when it comes to setting up each exercise in your workouts, you may prefer one type over the others. Of course, if you already belong to a gym with a decent selection of weights, you can move on to Part Two and get started. However, it is valuable to read on to learn how a few other pieces of exercise equipment will add variety and muscular improvement to your dumbbell experience.

Here are the three styles of dumbbells you'll see most often. You'll find all three types available in sporting goods stores, exercise equipment outlets, and over the Internet.

FIXED-WEIGHT DUMBBELLS

Just as its name implies, this style of dumbbell is one solid piece of metal that weighs a certain amount. Unlike some dumbbells that let you slide more weight on and off with weight plates, fixed-weight dumbbells are the ones you're most likely to see in health clubs and gyms, lined up on their elongated racks somewhere on a wall next to a mirror.

Strengths: Technically, these are the most convenient of the three types of dumbbells because you can just grab whatever weight you need to use and go. Instead of fumbling with collars and weight plates or trying to do the math in your head, you'll find that they are especially helpful when you make the mistake of choosing a weight that may be a little too heavy or too light and want to switch weights quickly.

Weaknesses: If you're looking to be able to choose from different sizes of weights as your muscles get stronger, you need variety. But variety with fixed weights can be costly and cumbersome for a lot of people. One problem with fixed dumbbells is simply having enough space to store them if you have more than a few sets (that's if you can afford that many). Owning a set of dumbbells that range from 5 pounds to 50 pounds (in 5-pound increments) can cost anywhere from $300 to as high as $2,500, depending on which brand and type you buy. And unless you find them aesthetically pleasing on your floor, you'll also need a dumbbell rack—which can run you an additional $150 to $250.

The reason fixed-weight dumbbells range in price is because they also range in the quality of materials. The cheapest brands are typically unattractive, cast-iron weights that look more like concrete than actual metal. Some higher-priced ones have vinyl, rubber, or plastic wrapped around them to make them look nicer and keep them from making as much noise when you accidentally clank them together. The higher-end versions are usually made from polished chrome. The good news is that no matter what type you can afford, your muscles won't know the difference because to them, weight is weight. More expensive doesn't mean better results—it just means they look nicer when you're not using them.

PLATE-LOADED ADJUSTABLE DUMBBELLS

This style of dumbbell is basically two handles that let you add or remove weight plates, depending on how much weight you need to use. Some versions hold the weight plates in place using clips and collars that slide on and off by squeezing them. Just be careful of the cheaper ones that require a mini-wrench to loosen, as these tend to strip easily, making the collars useless and dangerous over time. Some versions even have ends on the handles grooved like a screw, so you can place a collar on it and twist it into place once you've added your weight plates.

You can find ready-made sets that include a pair of handles and an assortment of weight plates that you can slip on easily. They start at around $60 to $80 for an 80-pound set (which lets you make two dumbbells that can go up to 40 pounds or one that weighs up to 80 pounds). If you need a pair that's heavier than that, it's easy enough to buy a few extra weight plates as you need them. If you're willing to dole out the cash, there are versions out there—like Ironmaster's Quick-Lock Dumbbell set, which is a 150-pound set—that allow you to build dumbbells ranging from 5 pounds to 75 pounds (average price: $430+).

You can also build your own set from scratch. The first thing you'll need is a pair of "standard handles," which can range in price from an average of $10 to $35. (There are higher-priced versions that have a few more bells and whistles like ergonomically shaped grips and cushioned handles, for example.) These types of handles work with standard weight plates—the ones that have a hole in the center that's about 1 inch wide. If you plan on using heavy weights, you may want to shell out the extra money for a pair of "Olympic handles" instead, which costs between $80 and $100. This style of handle works with Olympic-size plates—the style of weight plate with a much larger hole that's about 2 inches wide.

The second thing you'll need are the weight plates. You could buy them for both styles separately at any major sporting goods store. But remember, you'll have to buy four of whatever size plate (2.5 pounds, 5 pounds, 10 pounds, etc.) you decide on to create two equally weighted dumbbells—one of each plate on either side equals two plates. Two dumbbells total equals four plates! For standard-size and Olympic-size plates, the prices can range starting at 49 cents per pound and up.

The last thing you'll need are the collars that go on the ends of each bar to hold the weights in place. There are different styles of collars (if you're wondering why the prices range, that's because Olympic collars are more expensive than standard collars):

- **Spring collars.** They look like oversize paper clips, but these steel springs widen when you squeeze their ends and tighten when you let them go, making them easy to take on and off quickly (range $4 to $15 a pair).

- **Clamp collars.** Slide them on, then turn the attached handle on its side and the collar locks into place ($20 to $30 a pair).

- **Quicklee collars.** These collars slide right onto the bars and automatically lock in place. Releasing them only takes pinching them with two fingers ($12 to $45 a pair).

- **Spinlock collars.** These types of collars slip on, then you twist one or two screws to tighten them to the bar ($15 to $25 a pair).

- **Screw-on collars.** Each collar has a bolt on the side. Using a mini-wrench, you turn the bolt so that the end presses into the bar, keeping it firmly in place ($3 to $25 a pair).

Strengths: Because you can essentially change the dumbbell to weigh whatever you need it to, this option can be cheaper than having to buy a pair of weights for every size you plan to use. If you have enough weight plates to make a pair of 50-pound dumbbells, you essentially have enough to make 8 to 10 different-size dumbbells. They also take up less space than an entire rack of dumbbells.

Weaknesses: Using an adjustable dumbbell when lifting heavy weights can be a bit unwieldy because weight plates are long and thin and the heavier they are, the longer they are. Adding larger weight plates can make adjustable dumbbells too big so they aren't as comfortable to use for certain exercises.

The biggest disadvantage, however, is having to constantly dismantle each dumbbell every time you need to change its size. This can be especially frustrating when you're doing a series of exercises in a row that require different-size weights.

SELECTORIZED ADJUSTABLE DUMBBELLS

This new generation of dumbbell started back in 1991 with a product called the PowerBlock, and has evolved considerably since that time. To put it simply, this unique type of dumbbell lets you "select" the amount of weight you would like to use *before* you pick it up. A series of narrow weight plates all rest inside each other along each handle. Set the weight you want to use by either turning a dial, moving a pin, etc.—each brand uses a different method to change the weight—then simply pick up the dumbbell. It attaches only the amount of weight plates necessary, while the unused plates stay in the rack, letting you add from 5 pounds to as high as 130 pounds per dumbbell (depending on the model).

To keep the information in this book as relevant years from now as it is today, I won't get too specific with companies and their products, but there are a few that have been around long enough to justify the assumption that they'll be around tomorrow.

Bowflex SelectTech Dumbbells

These sleek selectorized dumbbells let you change their weight using a selector dial. Their version lets you adjust from 5 pounds to 52.5 pounds and retails for $399 (stand not included). (www.bowflexselecttech.com)

PowerBlock

The originators of selectorized dumbbells have up to eight different models now, with sets that go up to 21 pounds each ($129) to

45 pounds each ($250) to as high as 130 pounds each ($850). All it takes to change the weight is pulling out its selector pin, moving it up or down on the weight stack—depending on how many plates you want to add—then placing the pin back in to lock the weights in place—just like using a weight stack machine in a gym.

(www.powerblock.com)

Strengths: This unique style of dumbbell combines the space-saving freedom of adjust-

The *Other* Tools of the Trade

Now that you've picked your weights, there are a few other pieces of equipment you might consider purchasing. I know I told you that there are at least 4,988 possible dumbbell exercises in this book, but not all of them can be done using just dumbbells. To be fair, this is how all the moves break down—depending on what you have access to or feel like adding to your personal home gym.

- If you have only a pair of dumbbells, you can do 1,539 moves!
- If you have dumbbells and a chair, you can do 2,169 moves!
- If you have dumbbells and a flat bench, you can do 2,624 moves!
- If you have dumbbells and an incline bench, you can do 3,482 moves!
- If you have dumbbells and a decline bench, you can do 2,799 moves!

- If you have dumbbells and an incline/decline bench, you can do 3,657 moves!
- If you have dumbbells and a Swiss ball, you can do 2,644 moves!
- If you have dumbbells and a preacher curl bench, you can do 1,611 moves!

(Did you add up all these numbers and wonder why the total number is higher than the final number I gave you earlier? That's because certain pieces of equipment are more versatile and can be used to perform other exercises that may require a different piece of equipment. For example, if you have an incline bench, most recline into a flat position, which lets you also perform any exercise in the book that requires either a flat bench or a chair.)

FLAT BENCH BENEFITS

Nothing beats the support of a quality flat bench. You can sit on it, lie on it, even stand on it if necessary, which trust me you will, especially if you plan on trying every exercise in this book. Being able to lie back on the bench also allows you to lower your arms and elbows below your torso. This widens your range of motion for many moves, which forces more of your muscles to work than trying the exercise simply lying flat on the floor.

INCLINE-DECLINE BENEFITS

A normal flat bench keeps your shoulders in line with your waist as you exercise, which is still very effective but can be limiting to your body. The only way to forge a physique that looks great from every possible angle requires working your

able dumbbells without any of the inconvenience—since it takes only seconds to change the weight load.

Weaknesses: Its only major disadvantage: price. If you're just starting to weight train, you may not be prepared to invest that much money, whereas with fixed dumbbells or an adjustable set that you can make yourself, it's easier to buy what you need for cheaper—until your muscles demand a little bit more weight down the road.

muscles from every possible angle. That's why lying on an incline bench (where your shoulders are above your waist) or on a decline bench (where your shoulders are below your waist) can add significant advantages—and angles—to your workouts.

Just placing your body at an angle a few degrees off from what it's used to can switch which muscle fibers you fire as you exercise. It's a perk most intermediate exercisers rely on when working their chests, but these benches can help you intensify your workouts for any muscle group that uses exercises that require lying on a bench.

SWISS BALL BENEFITS
This unisex piece of fitness equipment is more than just some oversize inflatable ball. It's round and squishy for a reason. Whether you sit on it, lie on your belly, or lie flat on your back, it forces your body to spend more energy, coordination, and calories (not many, but a few) just to keep you from rolling off. It also teaches the muscles you're training—depending on the exercise—to work with all the tiny stabilizing muscles and microscopic nerves responsible for keeping your body balanced every waking moment of your day. That's why adding a Swiss ball to certain exercises can bring an extra stability advantage, if you're more performance-minded.

However, if overall size and strength is your goal, kick the ball in the corner. Sticking with exercises that aren't as challenging to your overall balance is much better for helping you focus all your energy on the muscles you're trying to shape and build—instead of sharing that effort with other supportive muscles that are working hard trying to keep you from falling over.

PREACHER CURL BENCH
I mention this piece of equipment here because one series of Master Moves (the Preacher Curl) is named after it. This specialty bench lets you sit down and rest your upper arms overtop the pad attached in front. This positions your arms at an angle, which makes it harder to cheat using your back muscles or momentum, so more effort is directed onto your biceps as you curl. But don't worry if you don't have one, or don't have access to it in your gym. I have six other ways you can perform the move without a preacher curl bench, along with many other variations you can try with all six to create even more unique dumbbell exercises.

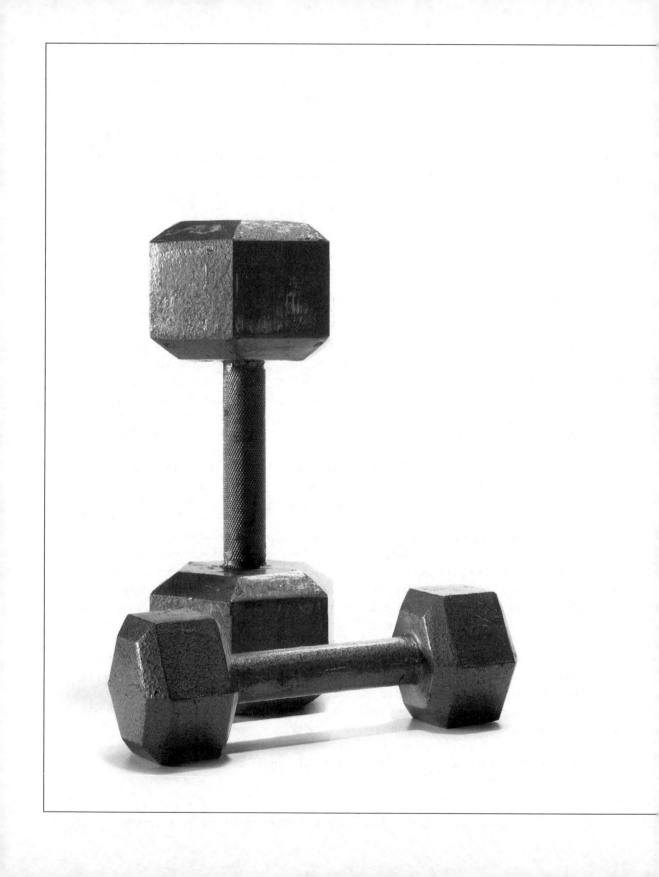

PART TWO

THE MASTER
MOVES

Four

GETTING STARTED

TOO MANY EXERCISE BOOKS make working out more confusing than it really has to be.

This book may contain 4,988 exercises, but by no means do you have to try them all. All you really need to do to build lean muscle, lose weight, and create that sculpted, chiseled look you've been striving for are the main exercises—known here simply as the Master Moves. These are the exercises that start each and every section in the next chapter. They're also the exercises recommended in all of the routines in the back of this book.

Still, it's nice to know that you have access to thousands of other exercises, if and when your mind and muscles decide they need a change of pace. That's why after you learn these basic Master Moves, you'll learn simple ways to spice each of them up with a few subtle tweaks. By making these changes, you'll stimulate your muscles in different ways so they continue to grow and develop in the way you're training for them. Which changes and tweaks you make will all depend on your level of exercise experience.

HOW IT ALL BREAKS DOWN

That's a lot of exercises to describe, isn't it? In fact, you probably have about as much interest in reading 4,988 exercise descriptions as I had in writing them. That's why this book uses a special system to maximize the volume of moves inside it—without wasting your time. A system that shows you the most effective dumbbell exercises for reshaping your body first, then teaches you how to multiply them into thousands of exercises to match whatever fitness goal you may have—no matter what your current fitness level may be.

STAGE ONE: SAY HELLO TO THE MASTER MOVES

In each section of the next chapter, you'll find a series of basic dumbbell exercises. These "Master Moves" are versions of specific basic exercises, such as shoulder presses, chest presses, biceps curls, and back rows, for example. These are the underpinnings of most of the thousands of exercises you'll learn about in this book.

Most experts would agree that you could easily build the body you've always wanted—and keep it that way for the rest of your life—using nothing but these classic, tried-and-true exercises. They may not seem as exciting when you're doing them, but to your body, they are the best ways to stress your muscles and stimulate their growth. But since variety is the spice of life, sometimes these Master Moves need a little tweak here or a subtle change there to breathe new life into an old routine. That's where the next stage takes over.

STAGE TWO: GET READY TO "MULTIPLY YOUR MOVES!"

After each group of Master Moves, you'll find a section called "Multiply Your Moves!" If the Master Moves are the main ingredients of your workout, the tweaks and tips in this section should be considered the spices you add to amp up the flavor of your workout. This is also where I start showing you how to take these Master Moves and turn them into thousands of different variations.

Before you start using any of these tweaks and tips on any of the Master Moves, you should already be familiar with all of the steps of whichever Master Move you're looking to upgrade. You'll still use the same steps as whichever Master Move you're looking to tweak—but replace whichever step is recommended in this section to create a variation of it—then perform the exercise as usual.

So why would you want to create thousands of other exercises—especially if the Master Moves I'm about to show you are so effective? Well, having thousands of different exercises to choose from is the best way to beat exercise boredom and make a workout seem fresh again. All it takes is a twist of the wrist or doing the exercise unilaterally to get a whole different experience from any of the Master Moves. In fact, recalibrating the Master Moves with a simple tweak can produce a better overall result by targeting muscle fibers that would otherwise never be activated. These tweaks can even add a benefit or two you may not expect, such as training certain muscle groups to work together so you simultaneously improve your sense of balance and core strength as you build muscle and burn fat.

BONUS EXERCISES: COMBINE AND CONQUER

Last, but certainly not least, many sections also have a handful of exercises at the end that offer an innovative twist. They combine the Master Move of that section with either a Master Move from another section or an entirely different exercise altogether. These "multistep combination exercises" not only allow you to train the muscles you typically target when you perform that particular Master Move and its variations but also allow you to train other muscles that never get a workout otherwise. This can help you save time by training more muscles collectively—instead of separately.

If you're wondering if any of the tips in the "Multiply Your Moves!" section will work on these combination exercises, the answer is maybe. If there is a way to incorporate any, I will let you know. Otherwise, simply perform the exercise as described and don't get too creative or you'll run the risk of injury. *(Note:* I personally recommend that you be at a level in your training where you're already using some of the intermediate exercises in your routines before attempting combination exercises because many require a more advanced degree of coordination.)

THE LEVELS OF INTENSITY

How will you know which Master Moves and variations are right for you? Easy, since both are divided into four categories: beginner, intermediate, intermediate "plus," and advanced. I recommend that you start experimenting with the beginner Master Moves and variations first, then decide as you go if you're ready to try some of the more advanced Master Moves and variations, based on the following criteria.

Beginner

If you're just starting to use dumbbells for the first time—or it's been at least 6 months since you've weight-trained and you're just getting back in the game—these are the exercises and variations designed for you.

Some people *hate* thinking of themselves as beginners and immediately skip anything related to the word, but remember this: *Just because these exercises and variations are recommended for "beginners" doesn't mean they are in any way the least effective or the easiest to do.* In fact, many of the beginner exercises are some of the more challenging exercises in this book.

That's because many of them are the basic moves that are considered to be the most efficient exercises for building quality muscle. Without a foundation, there is no house. Each of these beginning exercises is like the support beam your body needs to have in place if your intention is to rebuild yourself and your muscles. So take them seriously—and use them often—until you need to amp up your routine, of course.

Intermediate

Once you feel experienced enough using the beginner Master Moves and variations—which can take between 1 and 4 months of continuous training, depending on how often you exercise and how quickly your muscles adapt to using the beginner exercises—you can start adding a few intermediate exercises and variations to your repertoire.

Some of the Master Moves in this category change the angle of your body during the exercise. This redirects attention to other muscle fibers within the same muscles you're trying to shape for better overall results. Other exercises in this category allow you to sit down or kneel, which allows you to concentrate on the muscles you're trying to work instead of spending energy and effort maintaining your posture and balance. Regardless of which intermediate exercises you choose, your muscles will appreciate them. Adding these moves into the mix helps you train each muscle more thoroughly for results you'll see from every angle.

Intermediate "Plus"

The more experience you have with the beginner and intermediate Master Moves and variations, the easier it *should* be to perform all of them flawlessly. If you're at that stage—and you'll know when you're ready— you're probably in need of a few exercises that can keep your workouts from feeling like the same-old, same-old. That's where these intermediate "plus" Master Moves and variations can help.

All of the intermediate "plus" moves and variations are the perfect change-up to any routine because they all require at least one of these three factors (if not all three):

- Experience

- Concentration

- Coordination

To be honest, you may never need to use any intermediate "plus" exercises and variations because, quite frankly, the beginner and intermediate versions are much better if

you're looking for the best development of size, shape, and strength. But these more intricate moves require more concentration as well as increased effort from your muscles in order to pull them off, which makes them ideal for those exercisers looking for an athletic or performance edge. Even if you're not an athlete, but you're experienced enough to use them, these more-complex moves can be a refreshing change-up for your muscles when they need a new reason to start growing again.

Advanced

You'll find only a few exercises and variations marked "advanced" in this book. That's because I believe the word *advanced* should be attached only to exercises seasoned exercisers—exercisers who have been lifting weights safely for a long time—should try.

Frankly, the people with the best-looking bodies out there—including many of the models, athletes, and celebrities you may wish your body resembled—most likely built their impressive physiques using nothing more than beginner/intermediate exercises. Just like Intermediate "Plus" exercises, the advanced moves I've placed in this book are for those looking for an athletic edge or for something to make exercise more interesting again. But remember this:

Too many books allow their readers to "level up" and call themselves advanced after 6 months of training, then suggest exercises that their readers may not necessarily be ready to do. My aim in saying this is to help you avoid getting hurt trying something you're curious about but might not be conditioned enough to do. That's why I've reserved this term for Master Moves—and variations—that require a certain amount of exercise experience and your undivided attention when performing them. Without either, these effective yet difficult moves could increase your risk of injury if not done properly. All of the moves under this heading in the book are attainable but should be attempted only when you've spent enough time experimenting with the rest of the Master Moves and variations in this book.

Don't worry—you'll get there soon enough.

Five

EVERYTHING IN THE "RIGHT" ORDER

HERE IT IS. The chapter that pretty much makes up the bulk of the book. And if you use this book correctly, it's also the chapter that consists of the bulk of exercises you'll be using for a lifetime. Finding the exercises you need in a book of thousands may seem like more of a challenge than doing the exercises themselves. That's why this particular book is arranged in a way that makes navigating through it a bit easier than most.

MUSCLES IN THE "RIGHT" ORDER

In the back section of this book, you'll be instructed which exercises to do, depending on which routine you decide to use. But not everyone follows the best-laid plans. I fully expect you to eventually go off on your own one day and design your own workouts instead. That's why this book is arranged so you can find those exercises when you need them now—and when you'll need them later.

Many fitness books arrange exercises according to which muscles they work. The problem is after that, they simply place exercises in order of the most popular moves in the beginning with the least favorite exercises following up the lead. This arrangement can make it tricky, if not impossible, to find exercise descriptions quickly. They also tend to arrange the muscle sections in order from larger muscle groups to smaller muscle groups (chest, back, legs, shoulders, arms, and abs) instead of making it easier for the reader by placing them in alphabetical order (abs, arms, back, chest, legs, and shoulders).

EXERCISES IN THE *RIGHT* ORDER

This book also arranges exercises according to which muscles they work, but instead of throwing them in each category randomly, they're in alphabetical order. For example, there are 24 basic ways you can do a biceps curl in this book—each different than the next—but they can all be found under the "biceps curl" section, arranged according to their skill level. Within each difficulty level, they are also arranged in alphabetical order, making them much easier to find. Even the tweaks within the "Multiply Your Moves!" section are arranged in alphabetical order—making this a much smarter, faster approach to choosing the exercises you're looking for.

THE MAIN EXERCISES

Many exercises are surprisingly similar to each other, which is why I've arranged them in groups, according to whichever basic exercise. The main categories of basic exercises you'll find in this book are as follows:

- **BACK ROW** (works your upper and lower back)

- **BENT-OVER RAISE** (works your posterior deltoids—the back of your shoulders)

- **BICEPS CURL** (works your biceps—the front of your arms—as well as your forearms)

- **CALF RAISE** (works your lower legs)

- **CHEST FLY** (works your chest and anterior deltoids—the front of your shoulders)

- **CHEST PRESS** (works your chest, shoulders, and triceps)

- **CRUNCH** (works your rectus abdominis—otherwise known as your abs)

- **DEADLIFT** (works your entire back, legs, calves, abs, and gluteul muscles—otherwise known as your glutes or butt muscles)

- **FRONT RAISE** (works your anterior deltoids)

- **KICKBACK** (works your triceps—the back of your arms)

- **LUNGE** (works your legs, glutes, and calves)

- **LYING EXTENSION** (works your triceps)

- **PREACHER CURL** (works your biceps and forearms)

- **PULLOVER** (works your lower chest, triceps, and upper back, primarily the latissimus dorsi—the muscles that make up the sides of your back)

- **SHOULDER PRESS** (works your shoulders and triceps)

- **SHRUG** (works your upper back and trapezius muscles—the ones located between your shoulders and your neck)

- **SIDE RAISE** (works your medial deltoids—the sides of your shoulders)

- **SQUAT** (works your legs, glutes, and calves)

- **TRICEPS EXTENSION** (works your triceps)

EXTRA MOVES IN THE RIGHT ORDER

At the very end of each muscle group category, you'll find an additional assortment of exercises. These moves are just as important as the main categories of exercises that precede them. However, these exercises are more unique in their execution, which makes them impossible to place into any of the main groups I just mentioned. That's why they've been given a subsection all their own at the end of each muscle group section, arranged in alphabetical order, of course.

SOME FINAL POINTS TO KNOW
Where's the Word "Dumbbell"?

Because every single exercise in this book involves using a dumbbell or two, you won't find the word *dumbbell* in any of the exercise titles. A "dumbbell biceps curl" is simply called a "biceps curl," a "dumbbell triceps

extension" is simply called a "triceps extension," and so on, leaving more words to spend on even more variations and exercises.

When I Say "Light" Dumbbell, I Mean This . . .

In some exercises I will tell you to grab a "light" or "very light" dumbbell, instead of saying to simply grab "a dumbbell." When you see that in the exercise descriptions, try the exercise first with a dumbbell that's around 1 to 3 pounds to start. If that's too light, raise the weight in increments of 1 to 2.5 pounds and try again.

The reason you're asked to use a lighter weight than usual is typically because the smaller muscles you're working may not require that much weight to train. But remember: Just because I want you to use a light dumbbell *doesn't* mean it shouldn't be

The Main Categories

ABS
- Basic Crunch
- Additional abs exercises

ARMS
- Biceps Curl
- Kickback
- Lying Extension
- Preacher Curl
- Triceps Extension
- Additional arm exercises

BACK
- Back Row
- Deadlift
- Pullover
- Shrug
- Additional back exercises

CHEST
- Chest Fly
- Chest Press
- Additional chest exercises

LEGS
- Calf Raise
- Lunge
- Squat
- Additional leg exercises

SHOULDERS
- Bent-Over Raise
- Front Raise
- Shoulder Press
- Side Raise
- Additional shoulder exercises

heavy enough to exhaust your muscles by the end of your set.

When I Say "Heavy" Dumbbell, I Mean This . . .

A few exercises may instruct you to grab a "heavy" dumbbell or a pair of heavy dumbbells. If you're not training for strength or you're concerned about using heavier weights because of safety reasons, put your fears to rest. Most of the exercises requiring heavier dumbbells in this book are either moves that require little range of motion—so there's no danger to handling a heavier weight—or exercises where you'll be using more multiple muscles to perform the exercise (so the workload gets divided, trust me).

When you see that in the exercise descriptions, try the exercise first with a dumbbell that's a size you feel safe with. If it doesn't exhaust your muscles within the required amount of repetitions, try increasing the weight by 2.5 to 5 pounds and try again. Eventually, you'll figure out what weight is heavy enough to be considered heavy for you for *that* particular exercise.

EXERCISES FOR YOUR
ABS

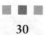

>>CRUNCH

This basic exercise strengthens and tones the rectus abdominis, one of the four muscle groups that compose your abdominals. However, performing this exercise in different ways can also target the other three muscle groups—your external and internal obliques, as well as the transverse abdominis. Note: Although the basic way to perform a crunch is without weights, this book is—after all—about dumbbells, so all of the versions you'll find in this section use one or two dumbbells in various innovative ways.

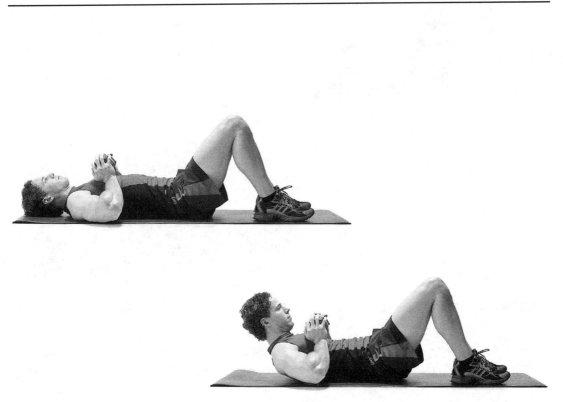

Basic Crunch

(WORKS UPPER ABS)

1. Lie flat on your back on a mat or carpeted surface with your knees bent and feet flat on the floor.

2. Grab a light dumbbell with both hands by its ends and rest it on your chest with your elbows sticking out to the sides and your hands facing each other.

3. Holding the dumbbell in place, slowly curl your head then your shoulders off the floor, using your abs—not momentum—as the catalyst for the movement.

4. Lower yourself back down.

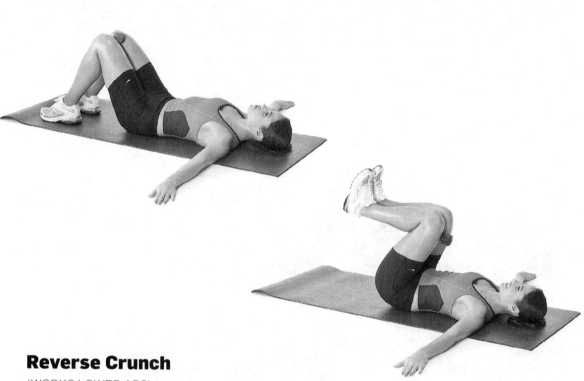

Reverse Crunch

(WORKS LOWER ABS)

1. Lie flat on your back on a mat or carpeted surface with your knees bent, feet flat on the floor. Place a light dumbbell between your thighs right between your knees and squeeze so it stays in place throughout the exercise.

2. Stretch your arms out to your sides—palms down—for support.

3. Holding the dumbbell in place, slowly curl your knees up to your chest, then lower your legs back down.

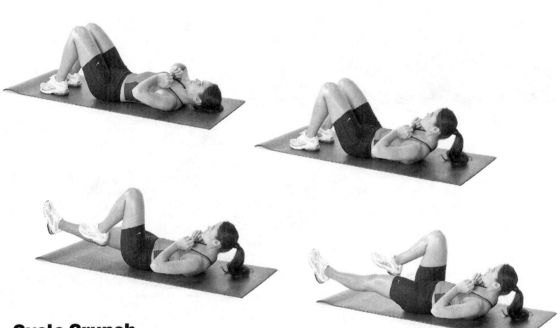

Cycle Crunch

(WORKS UPPER AND LOWER ABS)

1. Lie flat on your back—on a mat or carpeted surface—with your legs bent, feet flat on the floor.

2. Grab a light dumbbell with both hands by its ends and rest it on your chest—with your elbows out to the sides.

3. Holding the dumbbell in place, slowly curl your head and shoulders off the floor and stay in this elevated position.

4. Slowly pull your left knee in toward your chest as you extend your right leg straight out. Your right foot should be suspended about 1 to 2 inches off the floor.

5. Reverse the motion by extending your left leg as you slowly pull your right knee in toward your chest. Continue alternating between your left and right leg throughout the exercise.

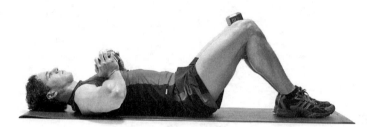

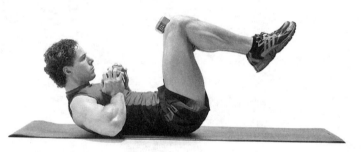

Double Crunch

(WORKS UPPER AND LOWER ABS)

1. Lie flat on your back on a mat or carpeted surface with your knees bent, feet flat on the floor. Place a light dumbbell between your thighs—right above your knees—and squeeze it so it stays in place throughout the exercise.

2. Grab another light dumbbell with both hands by its ends and rest it on your chest—with your elbows out to the sides.

3. Holding the dumbbells in place, slowly curl your head and shoulders off the floor as you simultaneously curl your knees up to your chest.

4. Pause at the top, then lower yourself back down.

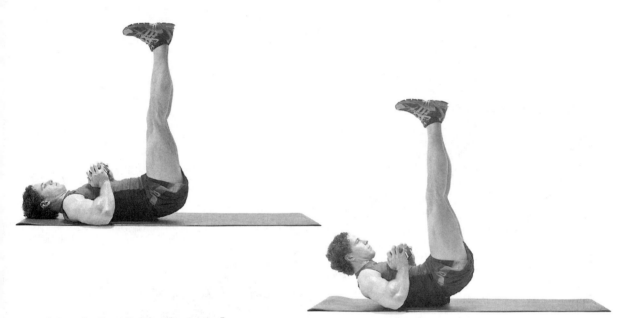

Straight-Leg Crunch

(WORKS UPPER AND LOWER ABS)

1. Lie flat on your back on a mat or carpeted surface and extend your legs up so that your heels are pointing to the ceiling.

2. Grab a light dumbbell with both hands by its ends and tuck it to your chest—elbows out to the sides.

3. Keeping your legs straight, slowly curl your head and shoulders off the floor.

4. Slowly lower yourself back down.

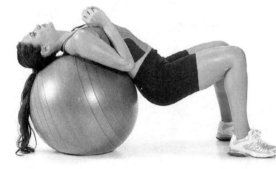

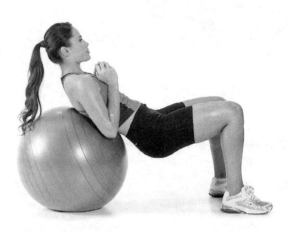

Swiss-Ball Crunch

(WORKS LOWER ABS)

1. Lie back on top of a Swiss ball with your head, shoulders, and back resting on the ball's surface—legs bent, feet flat on the floor.

2. Grab a light dumbbell with both hands by its ends and tuck it to your chest—elbows out to the sides.

3. Keeping the dumbbell held to your chest, slowly curl your shoulders and upper back up off the ball while concentrating on steadying the ball as you go.

4. Slowly lower yourself back down.

Multiply Your Moves! Beginner

Rotate Your Knees (creates 2 "new" moves!) Every time you curl your knees to your chest, pause at the top, then bend slightly at the waist and rotate your knees a few inches to the left, then rotate a few inches to the right. Bring your knees back to center and lower them back down.

Twist Left-Twist Right (creates 4 "new" moves!) Instead of curling your shoulders and upper back forward—up and down—try twisting to the left at the top of the move. Lower yourself back down, then lift and twist to the right for the next repetition. Continue to alternate from left to right for the duration of the exercise.

Multiply Your Moves! Intermediate

Press the Weight (creates 4 "new" moves!) Instead of keeping the weight held to your chest as you curl up and down, extend your arms as you curl up and raise the weight straight above you. As you curl back down, pull the weight back into your chest.

Extend Your Arms (creates 5 "new" moves!) Instead of keeping the weight held to your chest, extend your arms straight up so that the weight is held above you. Then, keep them extended above you as you crunch.

Multiply Your Moves! Intermediate "Plus"

Feet Elevated (creates 3 "new" moves!) Instead of keeping your feet flat on the floor—or touching them back down if you're doing any variation where you raise them off the floor—try suspending them an inch off the floor. This keeps continuous tension on the lower portion of your abs through-out the entire exercise.

Sweep Your Arms (creates 4 "new" moves!) Instead of holding the weight to your chest, hold the weight by its ends. Extend your arms back behind your head before you begin the exercise so that your upper arms are flush with your ears. As you crunch, slowly sweep your arms forward—elbows unlocked—so the weight ends up directly above you at the top of the move. As you crunch back down, sweep the dumbbell back down behind your head to the starting position.

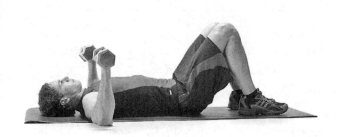

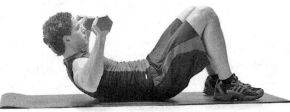

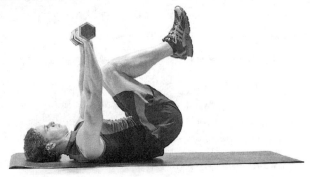

Press Crunch

(WORKS THE CHEST AND ABS)

1. Lie flat on the floor with your legs bent, feet flat on the floor. Hold a dumbbell in each hand and place them along the sides of your chest.

2. Holding the weights in place, slowly curl your head and shoulders off the floor.

3. Lower yourself back down to the floor, then pull your knees up toward your chest. Simultaneously press the weights up above you.

4. Lower the weights back down as you lower your legs back to the floor.

≫ADDITIONAL ABDOMINAL EXERCISES

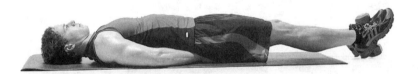

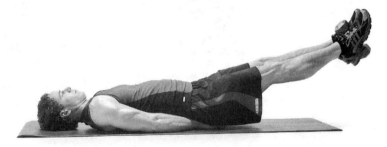

Dumbbell Leg Lift

(WORKS THE LOWER ABS)

1. Lie flat on your back with your legs straight. Place a light dumbbell between your feet (one end of the dumbbell should rest on the top of your feet with the other end touching the floor). Tuck your hands underneath your buttocks, palms facing down.

2. Keeping your legs together and your torso flat on the floor, slowly raise both legs up until your heels are about 12 to 18 inches off the ground.

3. Pause, then slowly lower your legs back down, stopping before the weight touches the floor.

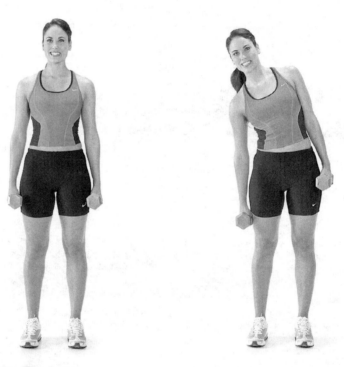

Standing Side Bend

(WORKS THE OBLIQUES)

1. Stand straight with a dumbbell in each hand, arms down along your sides.

2. Keeping your arms straight, slowly bend to the right as far as you comfortably can.

3. Return to an upright position, then bend to the left.

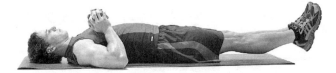

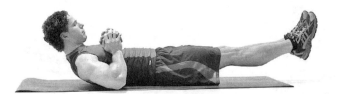

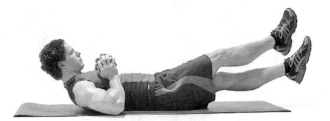

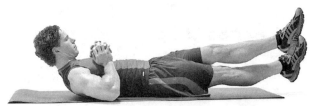

Scissor-Kick Crunch

(WORKS YOUR UPPER AND LOWER ABS)

1. Lie flat on your back with your legs straight—feet together—and raise your heels an inch off the floor. Grab a light dumbbell with both hands by its ends and rest it on your chest with your elbows out to the sides.

2. Slowly curl your shoulders up off the floor and hold this position.

3. Next, cross your left leg under your right, then alternate by moving your right leg under your left leg and hold that position.

4. Slowly lower your torso back down to the floor.

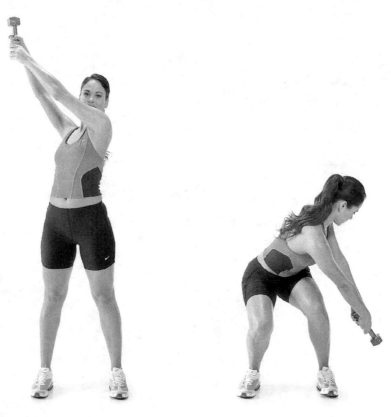

Weighted Chop

(WORKS THE ABS, SHOULDERS, AND LOWER BACK)

1. Stand straight with your feet shoulder-width apart and hold a light dumbbell with both hands around the handle like a baseball bat. Twisting at your waist, turn to your right and raise your arms overhead so that the weight is directly over your right shoulder—your left heel should rise off the floor as you pivot.

2. Starting from this position, squat down and rotate your torso to your left as you simultaneously "chop" the dumbbell across and down to your left.

3. When the weight reaches the outside of your left ankle, reverse the motion and return to the starting position where the weight is above your right shoulder. After the set is finished, switch positions so that you're twisting to your right—starting with the dumbbell over your left shoulder— and twist down and to the right.

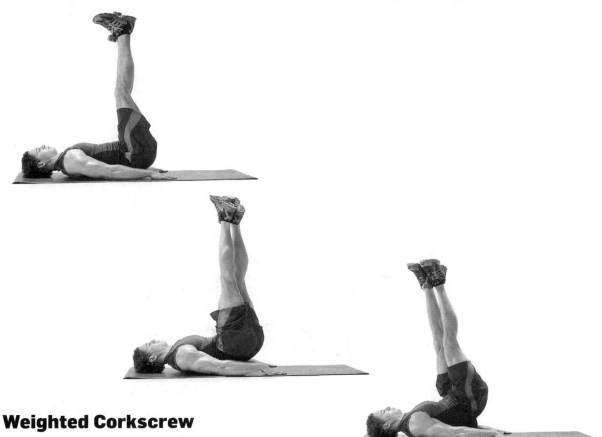

Weighted Corkscrew

(WORKS THE ABS AND OBLIQUES)

1. Lie flat on the floor with your arms next to your sides, palms flat on the floor for support. Straighten your legs directly above your hips so you look like the letter "L"—feet together with your heels pointing toward the ceiling. Have a training partner place a very light dumbbell between your feet.

2. Keeping your upper back, shoulders, and head flat, slowly raise your butt up off the floor and twist your hips to the left.

3. Lower your hips back down to the floor—keeping your legs straight and heels to the ceiling—and repeat the move, this time raising your hips up and to the right. Alternate back and forth from left to right.

EXERCISES FOR YOUR
ARMS

›› BICEPS CURL

This exercise works the biceps, forearms, and biceps brachialis.

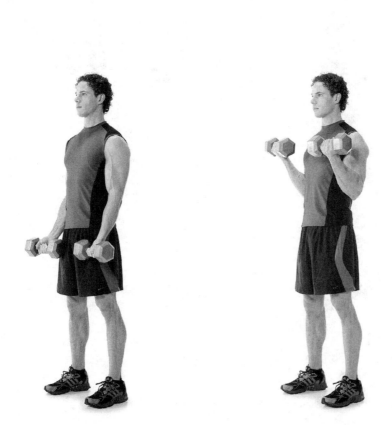

Biceps Curl

1. Stand straight holding a dumbbell in each hand, arms in front of you.

2. Turn your hands out so your palms face forward.

3. Without moving your upper arms, slowly curl the weights up until the dumbbells reach your shoulders—your palms should now be facing in toward your body.

4. Flex your biceps, then slowly lower your arms back down.

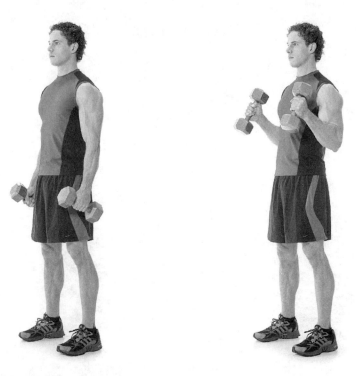

Hammer Curl

Keeping your hands locked in a neutral-grip position as you curl the weight up lets you incorporate the brachialis.

1. Stand straight holding a dumbbell in each hand, arms at your sides.

2. Turn your hands so your palms face in toward each other.

3. Without moving your upper arms, slowly curl the weights up until the ends of the dumbbells reach your shoulders—your palms should still be facing in toward each other.

4. Flex your biceps, then slowly lower your arms back down.

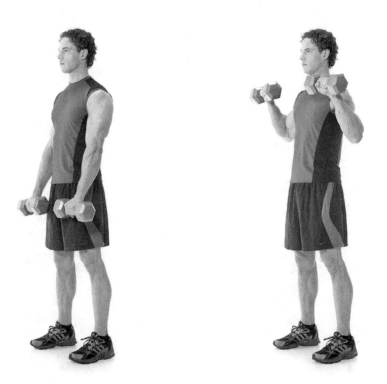

Reverse Curl

Keeping your hands fixed in an overhand grip throughout this exercise also works the brachialis, as well as more muscle fibers within your forearms. It also strengthens your hands because you have to maintain a tight grip on the dumbbells to keep them from falling as you curl.

1. Stand straight holding a dumbbell in each hand, arms in front of you.

2. Turn your hands in so that the backs of your hands face forward, instead of your palms.

3. Without moving your upper arms, slowly curl the weights up until the backs of your hands reach your shoulders—your palms should now be facing forward.

4. Flex your biceps, then slowly lower your arms back down.

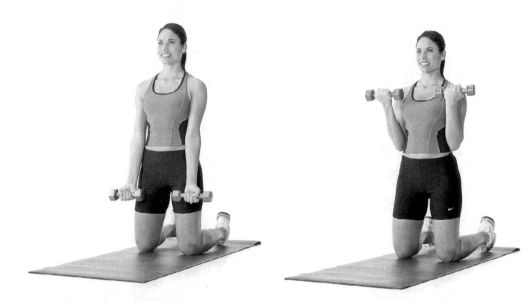

Kneeling Curl

Kneeling instead of standing makes it harder to use momentum to lift the weights, which places more muscle-building stress on your biceps.

1. Get into a kneeling position with a dumbbell in each hand, arms in front of you. Your back should be straight and in line with your thighs.

2. Follow Steps 2–4 of the Biceps Curl (see page 45).

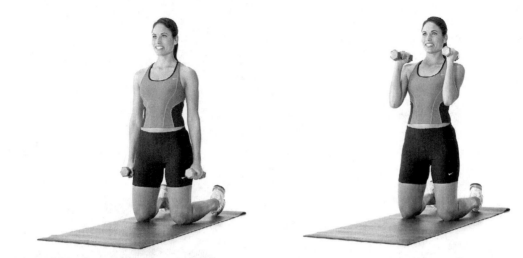

Kneeling Hammer Curl

1. Get into a kneeling position with a dumbbell in each hand, arms at your sides. Your back should be straight and in line with your thighs.

2. Follow Steps 2–4 of the Hammer Curl (see page 46).

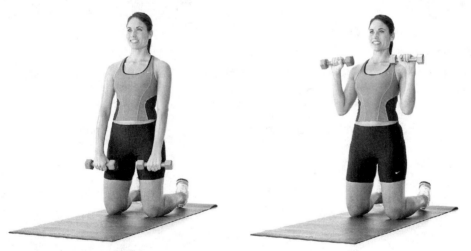

Kneeling Reverse Curl

1. Get into a kneeling position with a dumbbell in each hand, arms in front of you. Your back should be straight and in line with your thighs.

2. Follow Steps 2–4 of the Reverse Curl (see page 47).

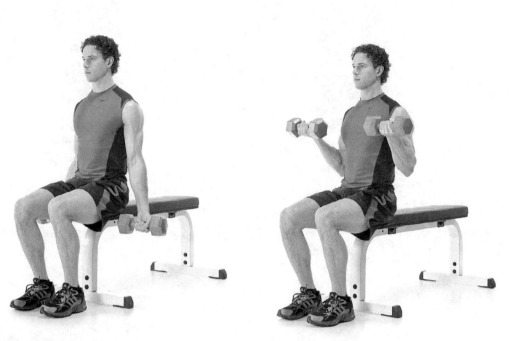

Seated Curl

Sitting down lets the bench help stabilize your body as you curl instead of your back and leg muscles, which occurs indirectly when performing the exercise standing. It also increases your range of motion as you curl without drawing help from your shoulders.

1. Sit on a bench—or armless chair—with a dumbbell in each hand, arms hanging down at your sides.

2. Follow Steps 2–4 of the Biceps Curl (see page 45).

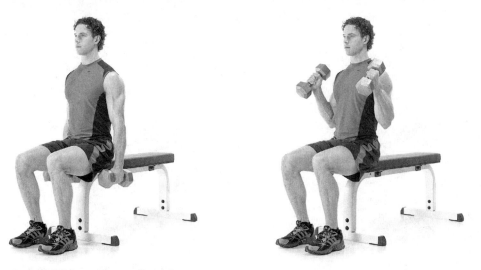

Seated Hammer Curl

1. Sit on a bench—or armless chair—with a dumbbell in each hand, arms hanging down at your sides.

2. Follow Steps 2–4 of the Hammer Curl (see page 46).

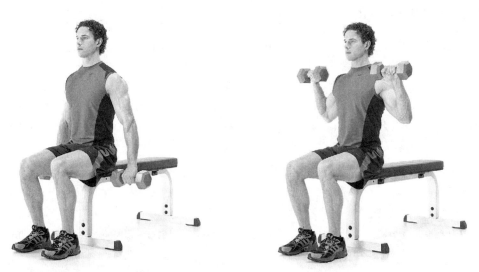

Seated Reverse Curl

1. Sit on a bench—or armless chair—with a dumbbell in each hand, arms hanging down at your sides.

2. Follow Steps 2–4 of the Reverse Curl (see page 47).

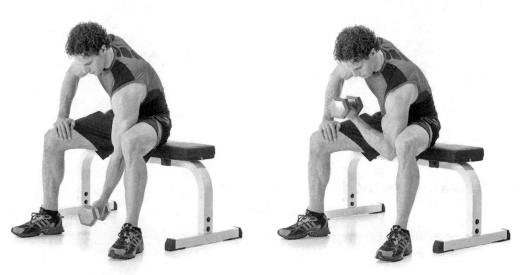

Concentration Curl

This variation lets you target each arm separately, while the position also eliminates cheating (if you don't lean back as you curl) so you can exhaust your biceps safely using less weight.

1. Sit on a weight bench—or chair—with your legs spread, feet flat on the floor. Grab a light dumbbell in your left hand and let it hang between your legs. Keeping your back flat, bend forward at the waist until the back of your upper (left) arm is pressed along the inside of your left thigh. Rest your right hand on your right knee for support.

2. Turn your hand out so your palm faces forward.

3. Keeping your upper arm tucked into your thigh, slowly curl the weight up until it reaches your left shoulder.

4. Flex your biceps, then slowly lower your arm back down. Repeat the set for the required amount of repetitions, then switch positions to work your right arm.

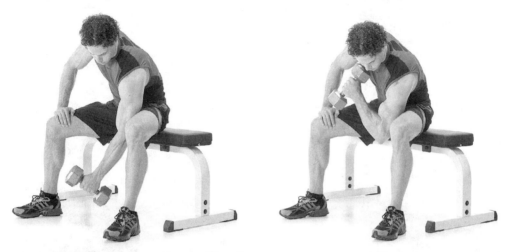

Concentration Hammer Curl

Follow the same steps as if performing a Concentration Curl (see opposite page), except Step #2. Instead of having your palm facing forward, rotate the weight in 90 degrees until the knuckle on your thumb is pointing forward.

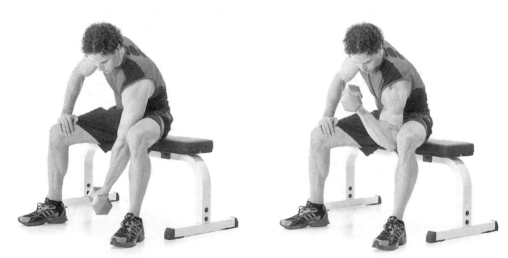

Concentration Reverse Curl

Follow the same steps as if performing a Concentration Curl (see opposite page), except Step #2. Instead of having your palm facing forward, rotate the weight in 180 degrees until your palm is facing backward.

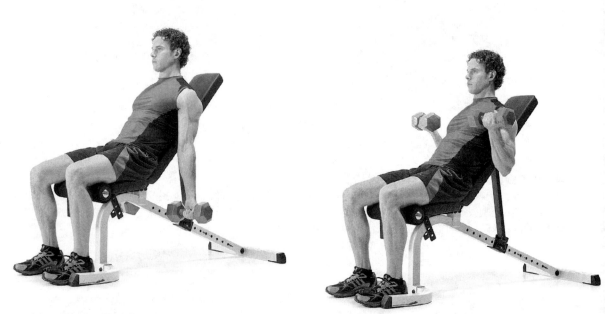

Incline Curl

Lying on an incline bench and letting your arms hang straight down angles them slightly behind your body instead of flush with your torso. This changes the effect of the move by redirecting the effort of the exercise to different muscle fibers within your biceps.

1. Sit on an incline bench with a dumbbell in each hand, arms hanging straight down—your arms will naturally fall slightly behind your body.

2. Follow Steps 2–4 of the Biceps Curl (see page 45).

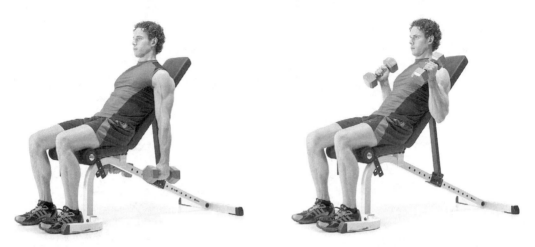

Incline Hammer Curl

1. Sit on an incline bench with a dumbbell in each hand, arms hanging straight down—your arms will naturally fall slightly behind your body.

2. Follow Steps 2–4 of the Hammer Curl (see page 46).

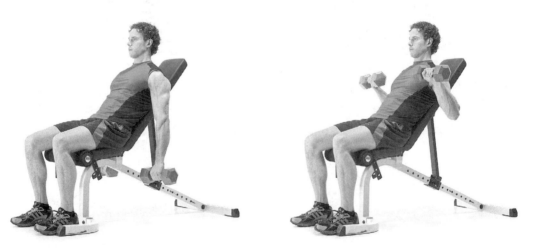

Incline Reverse Curl

1. Sit on an incline bench with a dumbbell in each hand, arms hanging straight down—your arms will naturally fall slightly behind your body.

2. Follow Steps 2–4 of the Reverse Curl (see page 47).

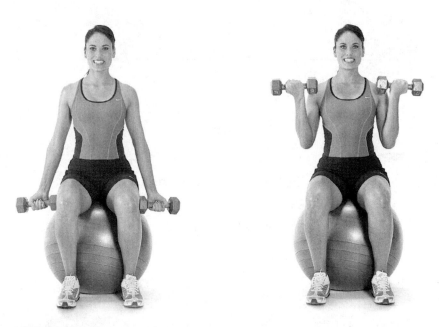

Swiss-Ball Curl

1. Sit on a Swiss ball with a dumbbell in each hand, arms hanging down at your sides.

2. Follow Steps 2–4 of the Biceps Curl (see page 45).

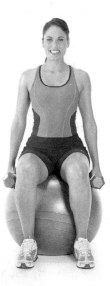
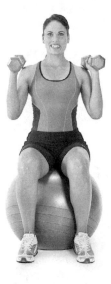

Swiss-Ball Hammer Curl

1. Sit on a Swiss ball with a dumbbell in each hand, arms hanging down at your sides.

2. Follow Steps 2–4 of the Hammer Curl (see page 46).

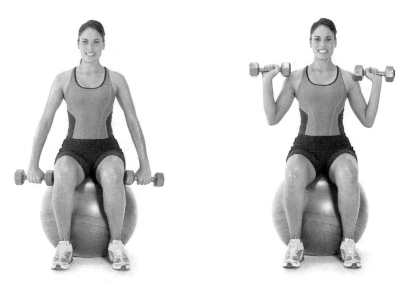

Swiss-Ball Reverse Curl

1. Sit on a Swiss ball with a dumbbell in each hand, arms hanging down at your sides.

2. Follow Steps 2–4 of the Reverse Curl (see page 47).

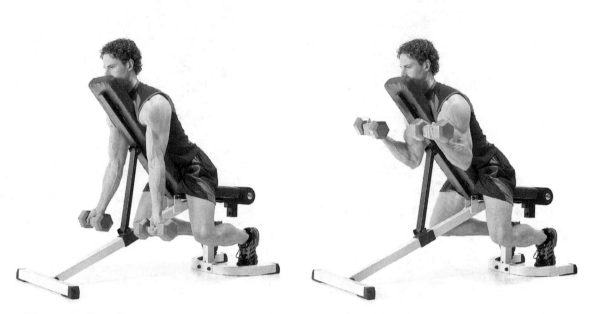

Prone Curl

This variation starts the curl with your arms slightly forward and away from your body. This helps to keep all the emphasis on your biceps by eliminating the first 15 to 20 degrees of the exercise—where most people tend to use momentum to get the weights off their legs and heading upward.

1. Set an incline bench at a 45-degree angle and grab a dumbbell in each hand.

2. Sit down on the bench so that you are facing the incline and rest your chin, chest, and stomach flat along the backrest of the bench. Let your arms hang straight down.

3. Follow Steps 2–4 of the Biceps Curl (see page 45).

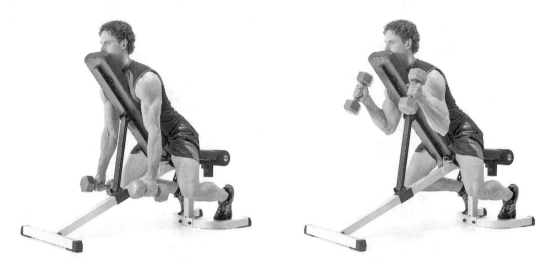

Prone Hammer Curl

Follow the same steps as if performing a Prone Curl (see opposite page), except instead of having your palms face forward, rotate the weights in toward your body 90 degrees until your palms face in toward your thighs.

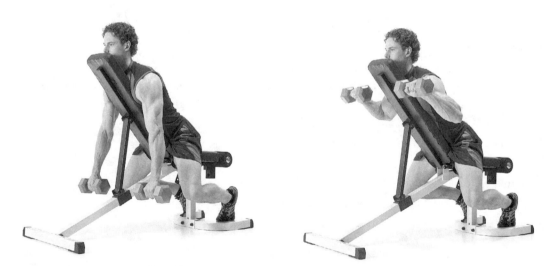

Prone Reverse Curl

Follow the same steps as if performing a Prone Curl (see opposite page), except instead of having your palms face forward, rotate the weights in 180 degrees so that your palms face behind you.

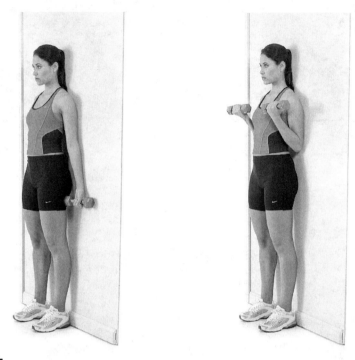

Wall Curl

Pressing your body against a flat, stable wall makes it virtually impossible to use momentum or any other muscles besides your biceps to curl the weight up. It's a perfect way to isolate your muscles, which is why you should start with a weight that's about 50 percent lighter than what you typically use when standing.

1. Stand against a wall holding a dumbbell in each hand, arms hanging down at your sides, feet shoulder-width apart.

2. Flatten yourself against the wall so that your head, back, triceps, and heels touch the surface. (All four should stay glued to the wall throughout the entire exercise.)

3. Follow Steps 2–4 of the Biceps Curl (see page 45).

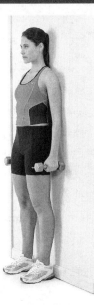 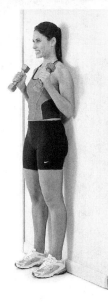

Wall Hammer Curl

Follow the same steps as if performing a Wall Curl (see opposite page), except instead of having your palms face forward, rotate the weights in toward your body 90 degrees until your palms face in toward your thighs.

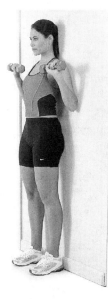

Wall Reverse Curl

Follow the same steps as if performing a Wall Curl (see opposite page), except instead of having your palms face forward, rotate the weights in 180 degrees so that your palms face the wall.

Multiply Your Moves! Beginner

There are 24 versions of the biceps curl in this section, but the possibilities don't end there. Adjusting all of them with these techniques can turn 24 exercises into 864 before your eyes.

Add a Twist (creates 48 "new" moves!) All three Master Moves—the biceps curl, the hammer curl, and the reverse curl—have you using a different grip (underhand, neutral, and overhand) for a reason. Holding dumbbells in these specific ways changes which muscle fibers you use when curling. However, you can still add a twist to each for a little variety—and to work more of your biceps.

For all eight of the Regular Curl variations: Start the exercise with your palms facing forward— but as you curl the weights up, either:

» Twist the weights in 90 degrees so your palms face each other at the top of the move.

» Twist them a full 180 degrees as you curl so the back of your hands face your shoulders instead. As you lower the weights, reverse the motion so that your palms face forward when your arms are back down.

For all eight of the Hammer Curl variations: Start the exercise with your palms facing in—but as you curl the weights up, either:

» Twist the weights outward so your palms end up facing your shoulders at the top of the move.

» Twist the weights in so the backs of your hands face your shoulders.

Regardless of which you choose, reverse the motion as you lower the weights so that your palms face each other when your arms are back in the starting position.

For all eight of the Reverse Curl variations: Start the exercise with your palms facing the wall behind you—but as you curl the weights up, either:

» Twist the weights outward 90 degrees so your palms face each other at the top of the move.

» Twist the weights a full 180 degrees so your palms face your shoulders instead. As you lower the weights, reverse the motion so that your palms face back when you reach the starting position.

Multiply Your Moves! Intermediate

One Arm at a Time (creates 24 "new" moves!) Instead of curling both weights simultaneously, try curling the weight in your left hand first. Lower the weight back down, then repeat the exercise, this time curling the weight in your right hand. Alternate from left to right throughout the set.

One Up, One Down (creates 24 "new" moves!) Instead of curling both weights together, curl the weight in your left hand first while keeping your right arm straight. As you lower the weight in your left hand, simultaneously curl the weight in your right hand. Continue the exercise by curling one weight as you lower the other for the entire set.

Curl and Lock (creates 24 "new" moves!) Instead of curling both weights together, curl the weight in your left hand first. On the way down, stop the weight halfway—so that your forearm is parallel to the floor—and freeze it in this position. Immediately curl the weight in your right hand up, then on the way down, stop your arm halfway and hold it there. Lower the weight in your left hand back down, then curl it back up and stop it halfway again before you fully lower it. Continue the exercise by curling one weight as you hold the other in a halfway position for the entire set.

Multiply Your Moves! Intermediate "Plus"

Push your arms even further by combining a beginner variation with an intermediate variation. These exercises definitely require more focus to do, but they can help you exhaust your biceps in a different way than your muscles may already be used to.

Add a Twist + One Arm at a Time (creates 48 "new" moves!) Try any of the 48 versions created by adding any of the six twists, but up the intensity by doing it one arm at a time.

Add a Twist + One Up, One Down (creates 48 "new" moves!) Try any of the 48 versions created by adding any of the six twists, but make it more of a challenge by curling the weight in one hand as you lower the weight in the other.

Add a Twist + Curl and Lock (creates 48 "new" moves!) Try any of the 48 versions created by adding any of the six twists, but lock one arm at a 90-degree angle—to keep tension on your biceps—as you curl the other.

Multiply Your Moves! Advanced

These small changes can make very big demands on your biceps by drawing different muscle fibers into the move, but they're not for anyone who's unseasoned. Try them when you're ready, but stop them if you experience any pain in your elbows or wrists.

Unbalanced Grip (creates 576 "new" moves!) Every exercise in this section—including all 264 variations—has you holding each dumbbell in the center of the handle so it stays balanced in your hand. Instead, try sliding your hand either all the way to the left or the right of the handle. Look down and your hands will look like one of these two positions:

» The thumb side of your hand(s) will be pressed against the inside plate of the dumbbell(s).

» The pinky side of your hand(s) will be pressed against the inside plate of the dumbbell(s).

The weights will feel off-center in your hands, no matter which way you choose to slide your hands. This unevenness forces your biceps to rely on different muscle fibers than usual to help balance the weight as you curl.

Weights In, Weights Out (creates 576 "new" moves!) Every exercise and variation in this section has you curling the weight up in a straight line. This keeps your hands spaced about shoulder-width apart. Here, keep your upper arms tucked into your body, but either:

» Bring the dumbbells closer together, so your hands are closer than shoulder-width apart, then keep them at that distance as you curl.

» Angle the weights away from each other slightly, so your hands are wider than shoulder-width apart, then keep them at that distance as you curl.

While having your hands shoulder-width apart develops your biceps best, widening your hands an inch or two recruits more muscle fibers around the inner part of your biceps. Bringing your hands in an inch or two recruits more muscle fibers along the outer part of your biceps. Note: This advanced tweak isn't easy to do for some concentration curl moves and variations, or when you twist both weights together. It depends on the size of the dumbbells you're curling and how wide your shoulders are. Instead, experiment first to see if Weights In, Weights Out feels natural when using it.

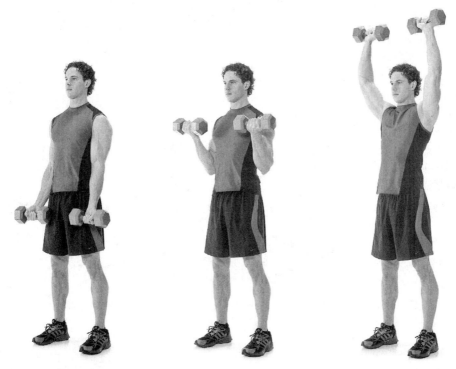

Curl and Press

(WORKS YOUR BICEPS, SHOULDERS, TRICEPS, FOREARMS, ABS, AND LOWER BACK)

1. Stand holding a pair of dumbbells with your arms down at your sides, palms facing forward.

2. Curl the weights up to your shoulders, then rotate the weights 180 degrees as you press them overhead. Your palms should face forward at the top of the move.

3. Reverse the move by lowering the weights back down to your shoulders, but don't twist them. Your hands should end up by your shoulders, palms facing forward.

4. Curl the weights back down until your arms are back in the starting position, twisting your wrists as you go so your palms face forward at the bottom.

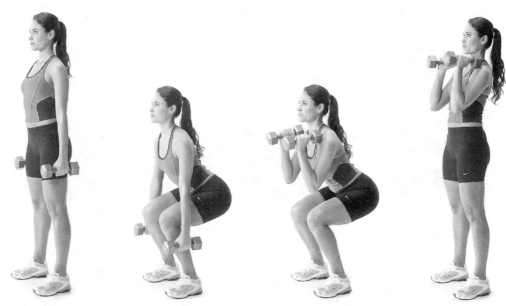

Curling Squat

(WORKS YOUR LEGS, BICEPS, AND FOREARMS)

1. Stand with your feet shoulder-width apart and a dumbbell in each hand, palms facing in.

2. Squat down until your thighs are parallel to the floor, making sure that your knees do not pass your toes.

3. Holding this position, slowly curl the weights up to your shoulders, but *don't* twist your wrists as you go—otherwise, the ends of the weights may hit your legs.

4. Stand back up and then curl the weights back down to your sides.

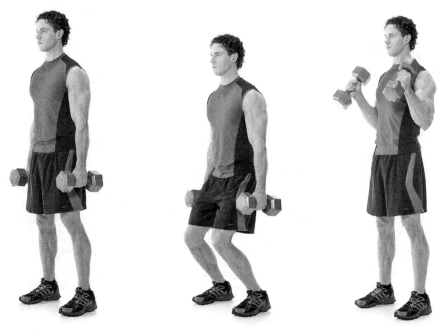

Push Curl

(WORKS YOUR LEGS AND BICEPS)

1. Stand with your feet shoulder-width apart and a heavy dumbbell in each hand, palms facing in.

2. Bend your legs and lower yourself down about 4 or 5 inches, then quickly push yourself up into a standing position as you curl the weights up to your shoulders. This allows your legs to help raise the weights with your arms.

3. Slowly lower the weights back down—taking at least 4 to 5 seconds to lower them.

≫ KICKBACK

This isolation exercise concentrates on building and strengthening all three of the muscles that make up your triceps—the lateral head, the long head, and the medial head.

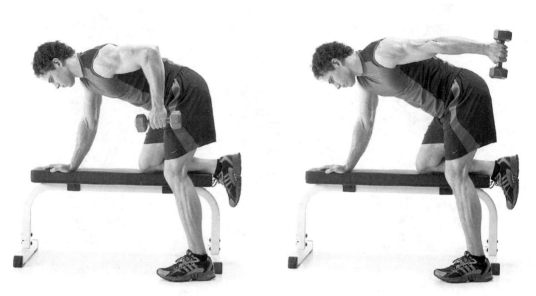

Basic Kickback

1. Stand with your right side next to an exercise bench—or the edge of a bed—holding a light dumbbell in your left hand.

2. Place your right hand and right knee on top of the bench, then bend forward at the waist until your torso is almost parallel to the floor.

3. Pull your left elbow up so that your upper arm is in line with your back. Your arm should be at a 90-degree angle, with your elbow pointing behind you, your knuckles pointing toward the floor, and your palm facing in toward your body.

4. Without moving your upper arm, slowly extend your arm out behind you until it's straight.

5. Squeeze your triceps, then bend your elbow to lower the weight back down. Finish the set, then switch positions to work your right arm.

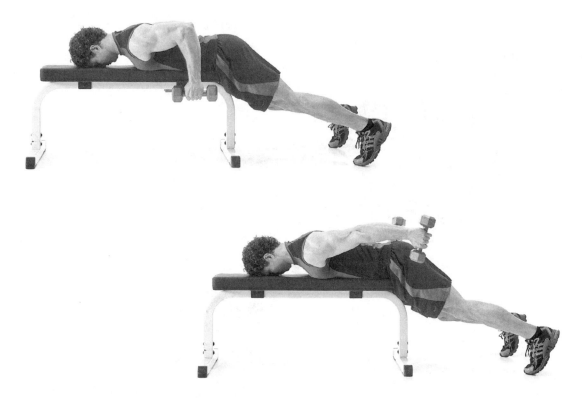

Flat Bench Kickback

1. Lie facedown on a weight bench holding a light dumbbell in each hand. Your legs should straddle the bench slightly—legs tucked in close to the bench with your toes touching the floor for stability.

2. Pull your elbows up so that your upper arms are in line with your back. Your arms should be at 90-degree angles, elbows pointing behind you with your knuckles pointing toward the floor—palms facing in.

3. Without moving your upper arms, slowly extend your arms out behind you until they're straight.

4. Squeeze your triceps, then bend your elbows to lower the weights back down.

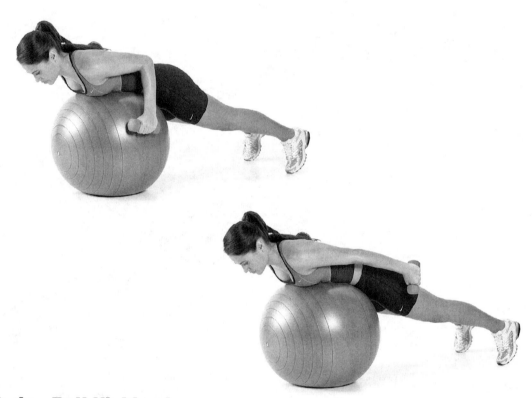

Swiss-Ball Kickback

1. Lie facedown on a Swiss ball holding a light dumbbell in each hand. Extend your legs straight out and place your toes on the floor—about shoulder-width apart—to keep the ball steady.

2. Follow Steps 2–4 of the Flat Bench Kickback (see page 69).

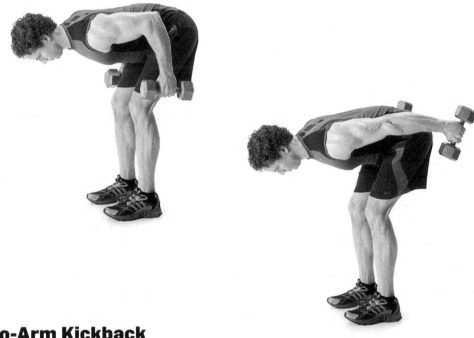

Two-Arm Kickback

1. Stand up straight with your knees slightly bent and your feet shoulder-width apart. Hold a light dumbbell in each hand. Keeping your back flat, bend forward at the waist until your torso is parallel to the floor.

2. Follow Steps 2–4 of the Flat Bench Kickback (see page 69).

Multiply Your Moves! Beginner

With only *four* effective versions of this isolation exercise to choose from, you can transform that number into 28 with these additional touches.

Underhand Grip (creates 4 "new" moves!) Before you start, twist your wrists so that your palms face forward. Then, keep them in this position as you extend your arms back—if you're using heavier weights, the end of the dumbbell may rub against your hip as you go. Use about 20 to 30 percent less weight than usual to start.

Overhand Grip (creates 4 "new" moves!) Twist your wrists so that your palms face backward. Then, keep them in this position as you extend your arms back—again, if you're using heavier weights, the dumbbell may rub your hip as you go.

Add a Twist (creates 16 "new" moves!)

If you're starting the exercise the traditional way—palms facing in—twist the dumbbells as you extend your arms either:

» Clockwise—your palms should face down toward the floor at the end of the move.

» Counterclockwise—your palms should end up pointing toward the ceiling.

If you're starting the exercise with an underhand grip—palms facing forward—twist the dumbbells clockwise 90 degrees as you extend your arms. Your palms should face each other when your arms are extended behind you.

If you're starting the exercise with an overhand grip—palms facing backward—twist the dumbbells counterclockwise 90 degrees as you extend your arms. Your palms should (again) face each other.

No matter which version you try, reverse the motion as you lower the weights back down so they return to their original position.

Multiply Your Moves! Intermediate

While these two variations don't apply to the Basic Kickback—since that exercise makes you work each arm separately—these tweaks apply to the other three variations that have you work both arms together.

One Arm at a Time (creates 3 "new" moves!) Instead of extending both arms, try extending one arm at a time, alternating from left to right throughout the exercise.

One Up, One Down (creates 3 "new" moves!) Instead of extending both arms together, try extending one arm first, then as you lower it back into the starting position, simultaneously extend the opposite arm. Continue the exercise by bending one arm as you extend the other for the entire set.

Multiply Your Moves! Intermediate "Plus"

Double your results by doubling up on your variations. Just combine a beginner variation with an intermediate move and add another 36 moves to your arm-sculpting repertoire. Just remember, these variations can't be used with the Basic Kickback.

One Arm at a Time + Underhand Grip (creates 3 "new" moves!) Before you start the move, twist your wrists so that your palms face forward. Then keep them in this position as you extend and lower the weights one arm at a time.

One Arm at a Time + Overhand Grip (creates 3 "new" moves!) Before you start the move, twist your wrists in so that your palms face backward. Then keep them in this position as you extend and lower the weights one arm at a time.

One Arm at a Time + Add a Twist (creates 12 "new" moves!) Choose any of the 16 versions created by adding any of the four types of twists, but do the exercise one arm at a time.

One Up, One Down + Underhand Grip (creates 3 "new" moves!) Before you start the move, twist your wrists so that your palms face forward. Then, keep them in this position as you extend one weight back as you lower the other arm.

One Up, One Down + Overhand Grip (creates 3 "new" moves!) Before you start the move, twist your wrists so that your palms face backward. Then keep them in this position as you extend one weight back as you lower the other arm.

One Up, One Down + Add a Twist (creates 12 "new" moves!) Choose any of the 12 bilateral variations created by adding any of the four types of twists, but make it more challenging by extending one arm as you bend the other back down.

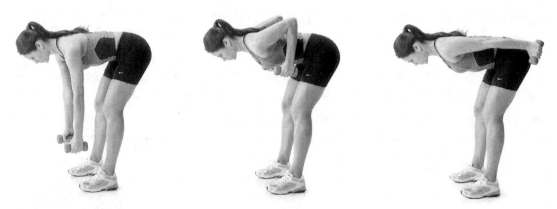

Row Kickback

(WORKS THE UPPER BACK, LOWER BACK, AND TRICEPS)

If you're game, you can use this two-part combo move for all of the variations in this section to create 14 new exercises. To demonstrate this two-part variation, I'll apply it to the Two-Arm Kickback.

1. Stand with your feet shoulder-width apart—knees slightly bent—and a light dumbbell in each hand. Bend forward at the waist until your torso is almost parallel to the floor, arms hanging down, palms facing in.

2. Row the weights straight up until they reach the sides of your chest and your arms are bent at 90-degree angles. Ideally, your upper arms should be parallel to the floor.

3. Immediately perform a typical kickback by extending your arms straight behind you.

4. Squeeze your triceps, then bend your elbows to lower the weights back down so that they are along your sides once again.

5. Finally, lower the weights back down until your arms are hanging straight down below your shoulders.

≫LYING EXTENSION

This exercise isolates the triceps—the muscles along the back of your arms. Because it focuses specifically on the three muscle heads that make up your triceps, this exercise doesn't require much weight to get the job done.

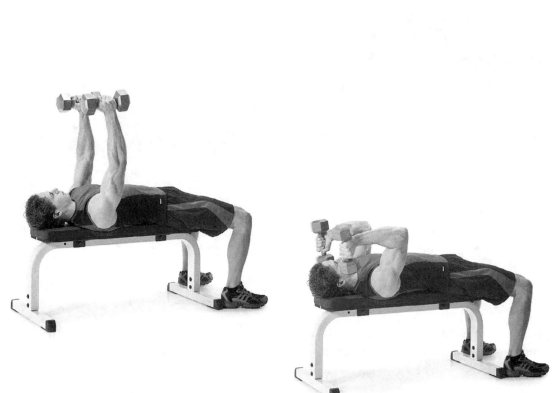

Lying Extension

1. Lie flat on a bench—or on the floor—with your knees bent and feet flat on the floor. Hold a set of light dumbbells in your hands.

2. Straighten your arms above you so that the weights are above your shoulders.

3. Turn the weights so that your palms face each other.

4. Without moving your upper arms, bend your elbows and slowly lower the dumbbells until they reach the sides of your head.

5. Slowly press the weights back up above you.

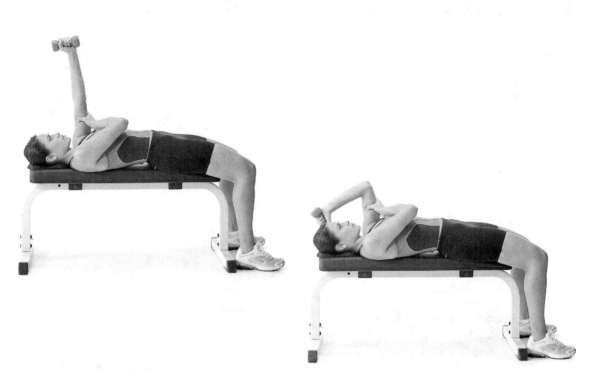

Lying One-Arm Extension

1. Lie flat on a bench—or on the floor—knees bent and feet flat on the floor—with a light dumbbell in your left hand.

2. Straighten your left arm so that the weight is above your shoulder. Reach across your chest with your right hand and cup the upper part of your left arm to help stabilize it.

3. Turn the weight so that your palm faces in.

4. Without moving your upper arm, bend your elbow and slowly lower the dumbbell until it reaches the side of your head.

5. Slowly press the weight back up above you. Finish the set, then switch positions to work your right arm.

Note: Don't let your upper arm move as you perform this exercise. At the start of every version of this exercise, point your arm up at the ceiling, then concentrate on fixing your upper arm in that place. The only body part that should move during this exercise is your lower arm as you bend your elbow and lower the weight.

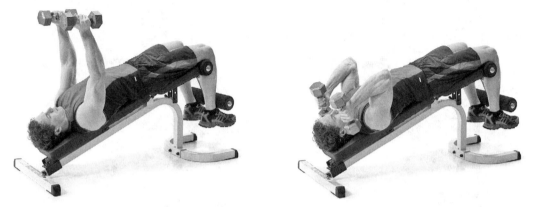

Decline Lying Extension

1. Lie on a decline bench set at an angle between 30 and 45 degrees below parallel with a dumbbell in each hand. Secure your feet at the high end of the bench for support.

2. Follow Steps 2–5 of the Lying Extension (see page 75).

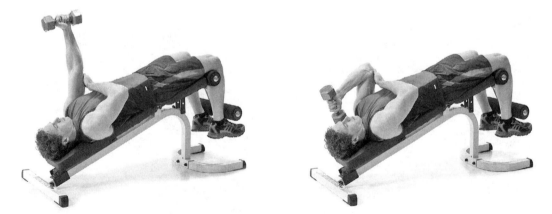

Decline Lying One-Arm Extension

1. Lie on a decline bench set at an angle between 30 and 45 degrees below parallel with a dumbbell in your left hand. Secure your feet at the high end of the bench for support.

2. Follow Steps 2–5 of the Lying One-Arm Extension (see opposite page).

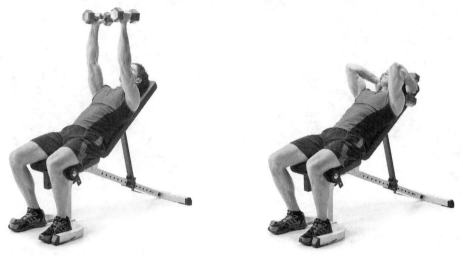

Incline Lying Extension

1. Lie on an incline bench with a dumbbell in each hand. Your knees should be bent with your feet flat on the floor for support.

2. Follow Steps 2–5 of the Lying Extension (see page 75).

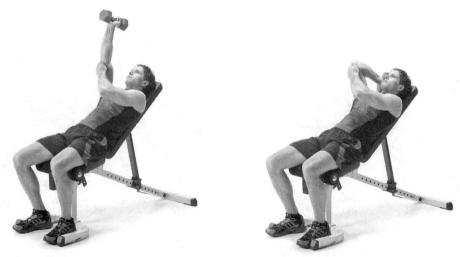

Incline Lying One-Arm Extension

1. Lie on an incline bench with a dumbbell in your left hand. Your knees should be bent with your feet flat on the floor for support.

2. Follow Steps 2–5 of the Lying One-Arm Extension (see page 76).

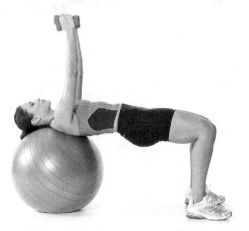 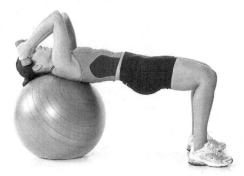

Swiss-Ball Lying Extension

1. Lie on a Swiss ball with your knees bent and feet flat on the floor with a dumbbell in each hand. Just your head, shoulders, and neck should touch the top of the ball—your lower back shouldn't touch it. Push your hips up so that your torso and thighs form a straight line—parallel to the floor—with your legs bent at 90 degrees.

2. Follow Steps 2–5 of the Lying Extension (see page 75).

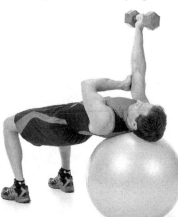 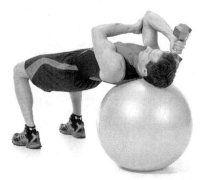

Swiss-Ball Lying One-Arm Extension

1. Lie on a Swiss ball with your knees bent and feet flat on the floor and a light dumbbell in one hand. Just your head, shoulders, and neck should touch the top of the ball—your lower back shouldn't touch it. Push your hips up so that your torso and thighs form a straight line—parallel to the floor—with your legs bent at 90 degrees.

2. Follow Steps 2–5 of the Lying One-Arm Extension (see page 76).

Multiply Your Moves! Beginner

There are *eight* different versions of the lying extension to choose from in this section, but you can pull off at least 68 other versions with these simple steps.

Every version of the lying extension has you keeping your palms facing in toward each other. Here are two tweaks you can apply to any exercise in this section, not just for variety's sake: Each of these changes redirects some of the effort onto different muscle fibers within your triceps. By mixing things up, your muscles get a more thorough workout so they can reach their full potential even faster.

Overhand Grip (creates 8 "new" moves!) Before you start, twist your wrist(s) so that your palms face forward—when you look up, you'll see the backs of your hands. Then, keep them in this position as you lower the weights down to your head and press them back up.

Add a Twist (creates 16 "new" moves!)

>> If you start the exercise in the traditional way with your palm(s) facing in, try twisting your wrist(s) in as you lower the weight(s) so that your palms face up when the weights reach your head.

>> If you start the exercise using an overhand grip with your palms facing forward, try twisting your wrists outward as you go so your palms face in toward each other when the weights reach your ears.

Whichever version you use, reverse the motion as you press the weights back up so your palms end up in the same position as they started.

Two Hands-One Dumbbell (creates 4 "new" moves!) Pick a heavier dumbbell than you usually use when doing a one-arm extension, but this time hold it with both hands instead of one hand. To get into position . . .

1. Rest one end of the dumbbell on your chest with the other end pointing up. Wrap your thumbs and forefingers around the handle and slide your hands up until your palms are flat against the inside plate of the end pointing up. Grab the weight tightly with both hands, then press it above you until your arms are straight.

2. Without moving your upper arms, bend your elbows and lower the weight behind your head.

3. Extend your arms back up until your arms are straight.

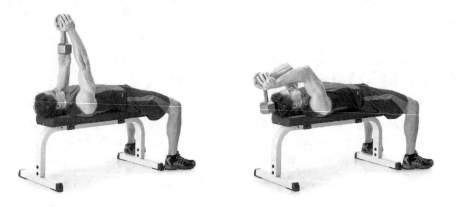

Multiply Your Moves! Intermediate

SINGLE-ARM EXERCISES ONLY

Cross-Shoulder (creates 4 "new" moves!) Holding just one weight instead of two gives you a little more breathing room in front of your face to try a variation that redirects more attention to all three heads of your triceps.

Instead of lowering the weight toward your head, lower the weight to the side so the dumbbell touches the shoulder of your opposite arm—your palm will face your chest at the bottom of the move. Simply reverse the motion to straighten your arm back up above you.

TWO-HAND EXERCISES ONLY

All four versions of the lying extension—where you hold *two* dumbbells instead of one—have you lowering both weights simultaneously. Try these two variations to mix things up a bit.

One Arm at a Time (creates 4 "new" moves!) Instead of lowering both weights, try lowering the weight in your left hand first, keeping your right arm pointing straight up as you go. Raise the weight back up, then keep your left arm pointing straight up as you lower the weight in your right hand. Alternate from left to right arm, for the entire set.

One Up, One Down (creates 4 "new" moves!) Instead of lowering both weights, try lowering the weight in your left hand first, keeping your right arm pointing straight up as you go. As you raise the weight back up, simultaneously lower the weight in your right hand. Continue the exercise by lowering one weight as you raise the other for the entire set.

Multiply Your Moves! Intermediate "Plus"

Which variations you try when you have some experience under your belt depends on whether you're looking to modify a one-arm variation or a two-arm variation. Either way, these hybrid exercises are truly challenging.

SINGLE-ARM EXERCISES ONLY

Overhand Grip + Cross-Shoulder (creates 4 "new" moves!) Before you start, twist your wrist so that your palm faces forward. Then lower the weight to the side toward your opposite shoulder—your thumb should end up pointing down.

Add a Twist + Cross-Shoulder (creates 8 "new" moves!)

» If you're starting with a traditional grip with your palm facing in, twist your wrist in as you lower the weight toward your opposite shoulder—your thumb should end up pointing down.

» If you're starting with an overhand grip—palm facing forward—twist your wrist out as you lower the weight toward your opposite shoulder—your palm should end up pointing down.

Multiply Your Moves! Intermediate "Plus"—*Continued*

TWO-HAND EXERCISES ONLY

Overhand Grip + One Arm at a Time (creates 4 "new" moves!) Before you start, twist your wrists so that your palms face forward. Then keep them in this position as you lower and raise the weights one arm at a time.

Add a Twist + One Arm at a Time (creates 8 "new" moves!)

» If you start the exercise in the traditional way with your palms facing in, lower the weight in your left hand first, keeping your right arm extended above you. Twist your wrist in as you lower it so that your palm faces up when the weight reaches your head. Reverse the motion as you extend your arm back up, then repeat with your right arm.

» If you start the exercise using an overhand grip with your palms facing forward, lower the weight in your left hand first while you keep your right arm extended above you. Twist your wrist out as you lower it so that your palm faces in toward your ear when the weight reaches your head. Reverse the motion as you extend your arm back up, then repeat with your right arm.

Whichever version you use, reverse the motion as you press the weights back up so your palms end up in the same position as they started.

Overhand Grip + One Up, One Down (creates 4 "new" moves!) Before you start, twist your wrists so that your palms face forward. To make it more challenging, lower the weight in one hand as you extend the weight in the other.

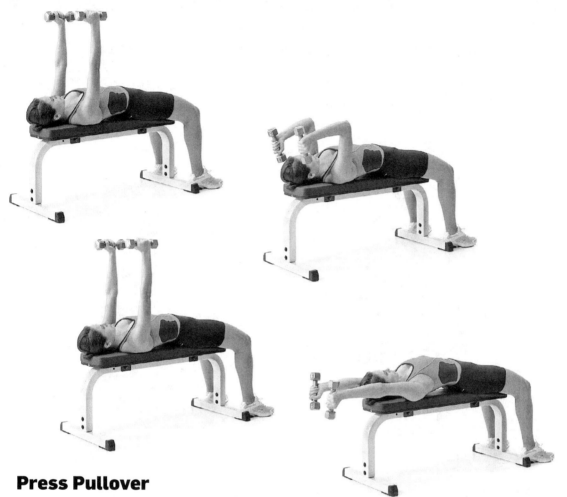

Press Pullover

(WORKS THE CHEST, SHOULDERS, AND TRICEPS)

1. Lie flat on a bench—or on the floor—with your knees bent and feet flat on the floor. Hold a light dumbbell in each hand and raise them over your shoulders, palms facing each other.

2. Without moving your upper arms, bend your elbows and slowly lower the dumbbells until they reach the sides of your head. Then press the weights back up above you.

3. Next, keeping your arms straight, elbows unlocked, sweep the weights back behind your head as far as is comfortable—your upper arms should end up alongside your ears.

4. Reverse the motion by sweeping your arms forward—keeping them fixed as you go—until the weights are back over your head.

>>PREACHER CURL

This biceps builder isolates your muscles by removing most of the momentum of the average biceps curl.

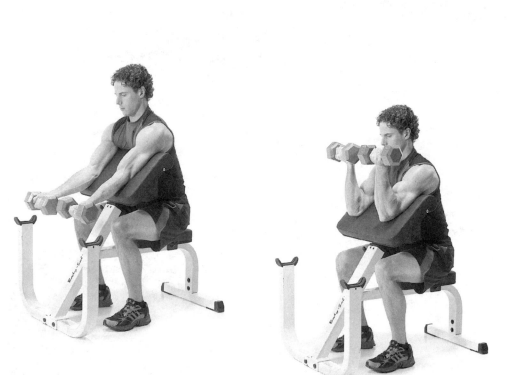

Preacher Curl

1. Grab a pair of light dumbbells and sit at a preacher-curl station.

2. Rest your upper arms on the slanted pad with your arms extended straight in front of you.

3. Turn your hands so that your palms face up.

4. Keeping your back straight, slowly curl the weights up until they reach your shoulders—your palms should now face the front of your shoulders.

5. Flex your biceps, then slowly lower the weights back down.

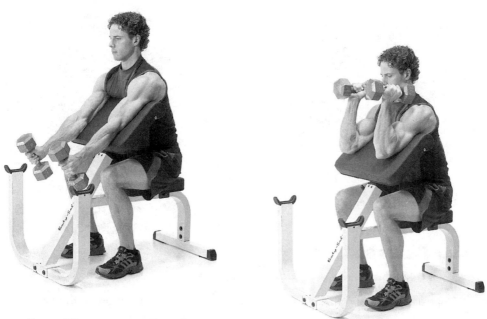

Preacher Hammer Curl

1. Grab a pair of light dumbbells and sit at a preacher-curl station.

2. Rest your upper arms on the slanted pad with your arms extended straight in front of you.

3. Turn the weights so your palms face each other.

4. Keeping your back straight, slowly curl the weights up until they reach your shoulders—the ends of the dumbbells should be facing your shoulders.

5. Flex your biceps, then slowly lower the weights back down.

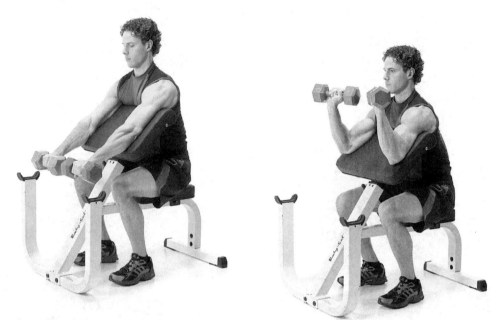

Preacher Reverse Curl

1. Grab a pair of light dumbbells and sit at a preacher-curl station.

2. Rest your upper arms on the slanted pad with your arms extended straight in front of you.

3. Turn the weights so that your palms face down.

4. Keeping your back straight, slowly curl the weights up until they reach your shoulders—the backs of your hands should end up facing your shoulders.

5. Flex your biceps, then slowly lower the weights back down.

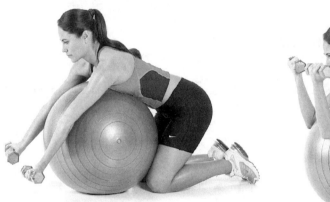 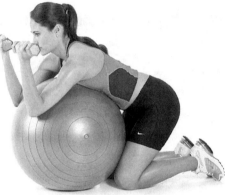

Swiss-Ball Preacher Curl

1. Kneel behind a Swiss ball with a dumbbell in each hand.

2. Extend your arms over the top of the ball and let your upper arms rest comfortably on the surface.

3. Follow Steps 3–5 of the Preacher Curl (see page 84).

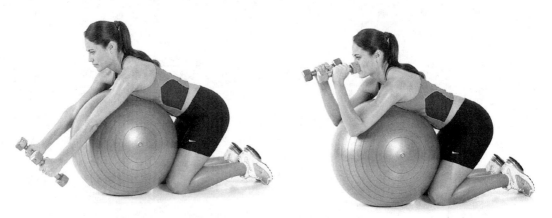

Swiss-Ball Preacher Hammer Curl

1. Kneel behind a Swiss ball with a dumbbell in each hand.

2. Extend your arms over the top of the ball and let your upper arms rest comfortably on the surface.

3. Follow Steps 3–5 of the Preacher Hammer Curl (see page 85).

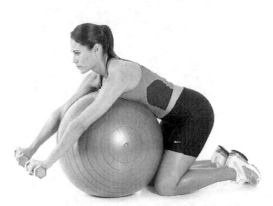

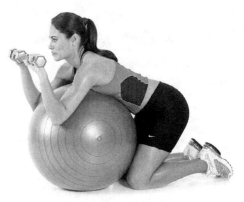

Swiss-Ball Preacher Reverse Curl

1. Kneel behind a Swiss ball with a dumbbell in each hand.

2. Extend your arms over the top of the ball and let your upper arms rest comfortably on the surface.

3. Follow Steps 3–5 of the Preacher Reverse Curl (see page 86).

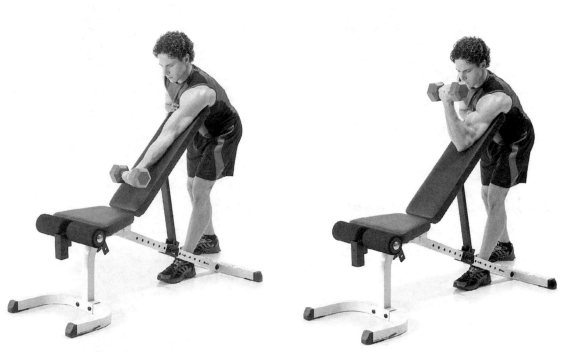

Incline Bench Preacher Curl

1. Set an incline bench so that the backrest is on a 55- to 65-degree angle—zero being flat and 90 degrees being perpendicular to the floor—then stand behind it with a dumbbell in your left hand.

2. Extend your left arm over the bench so it lies flat against it and your left armpit rests on the top of the bench. Your right arm can grab the side of the bench or rest anywhere that is comfortable so long as you are not using it for additional leverage.

3. Follow Steps 3–5 of the Preacher Curl (see page 84)—curling only your left arm for one set. Then switch positions and repeat the exercise with your right arm.

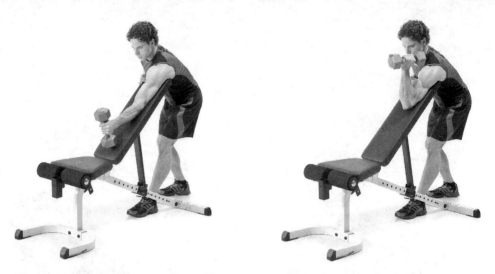

Incline Bench Preacher Hammer Curl

Follow the same steps for this exercise as you would when performing an Incline Bench Preacher Curl (see page 89), except instead of having your palm face up, rotate the weight in 90 degrees until your palm faces out to the side instead.

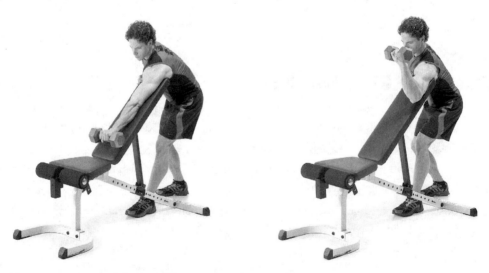

Incline Bench Preacher Reverse Curl

Follow the same steps for this exercise as you would when performing an Incline Bench Preacher Curl (see page 89), except instead of having your palm face up, rotate the weight in 180 degrees so your palm is flat on the bench at the start of the move.

Multiply Your Moves! Beginner

There are *nine* different versions of the preacher curl in this section, but 180 other variations are possible if you need to mix up the muscles you're exercising.

One Arm at a Time (creates 6 "new" moves!) Instead of curling both weights simultaneously, try curling the weight in your left hand first. Lower the weight back down, then repeat the exercise, this time curling the weight in your right hand. Alternate from left to right throughout the set.

One Up, One Down (creates 6 "new" moves!) Instead of curling both weights together, try curling the weight in your left hand first while keeping your right arm straight. As you lower the weight in your left hand, simultaneously curl the weight in your right hand. Continue the exercise by curling one weight as you lower the other for the entire set.

Multiply Your Moves! Intermediate

Add a Twist (creates 18 "new" moves!) All three curls—the preacher curl, the preacher hammer curl, and the preacher reverse curl—instruct you to use a specific grip (underhand, neutral, and overhand). Instead, try turning your wrists as you curl to engage even more of your biceps.

For all three of the Preacher Curl versions: Start the exercise with your palms facing up—but as you curl the weights up, either:

>> Twist the weights in 90 degrees so your palms face each other at the top of the move.

>> Twist them a full 180 degrees as you curl so the backs of your hands face your shoulders instead.

As you lower the weights, reverse the motion so that your palms face up when your arms return to the starting position.

For all three of the Preacher Hammer Curl versions: Start the exercise with your palms facing in—but as you curl the weights up, either:

>> Twist the weights outward so your palms end up facing your shoulders at the top of the move.

>> Twist the weights in so the backs of your hands face your shoulders.

Reverse the motion as you lower the weights so that your palms face each other when your arms are back down.

For all three of the Preacher Reverse Curl versions: Start the exercise with your palms facing down—but as you curl the weights up, either:

>> Twist the weights outward 90 degrees so your palms face each other at the top of the move.

>> Twist them a full 180 degrees so your palms face your shoulders instead. As you lower the weights, reverse the motion so that your palms face down when your arms are down.

Multiply Your Moves! Intermediate "Plus"

These two tweaks may not seem that difficult—since they're simply a mix of some of the beginner and intermediate variations you've already learned in this section. However, combining several into one move requires a greater amount of concentration and coordination that increases the level of intensity. Do these variations slowly, as they take a lot of attention to perform properly.

Add a Twist + One Arm at a Time (creates 12 "new" moves!) Try any of the 12 versions created by adding any of the six twists, but up the intensity by doing it one arm at a time.

Add a Twist + One Up, One Down (creates 12 "new" moves!) Try any of the 12 versions created by adding any of the six twists, but make it more challenging by curling the weight in one hand as you lower the weight in the other.

Multiply Your Moves! Advanced

This stability-challenging tweak can really surprise your biceps, but don't use it if you experience any pain in your elbows or wrists.

Unbalanced Grip (creates 126 "new" moves!) Every exercise and variation in this section has you holding the dumbbell(s) in the center of the handle. Instead, try sliding your hands either all the way to the left or right of the handle. Look down and either:

» The thumb side of your hand(s) will be pressed against the inside plate of the dumbbell(s).

» The pinky side of your hand(s) will be pressed against the inside plate of the dumbbell(s).

The weights will feel off-center in your hands, no matter which way you choose to slide your hands. This unevenness forces your biceps to rely on different muscle fibers than usual to help balance the weight as you curl.

>>TRICEPS EXTENSION

This exercise is similar to the lying extension, but positioning yourself upright as you perform the exercise works your triceps from a different angle that allows you to recruit more muscle fibers and lift more weight.

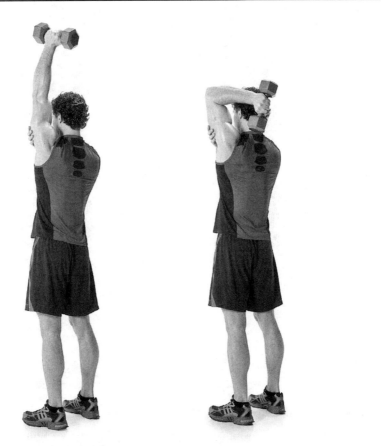

Basic One-Arm Extension

1. Stand straight with your feet shoulder-width apart, holding a light dumbbell in your left hand.

2. Press the dumbbell over your head so that your left arm is straight—palm pointing out to the side. Reach your right arm across your face and cup your left elbow with your right hand—this will help keep your upper arm stable as you perform the exercise.

3. Without moving your upper arm, slowly bend your left elbow and lower the dumbbell behind your head as far as possible.

4. Extend the dumbbell back overhead until your left arm is straight and repeat for one set. Then place the dumbbell in your right hand and repeat the exercise with your right arm.

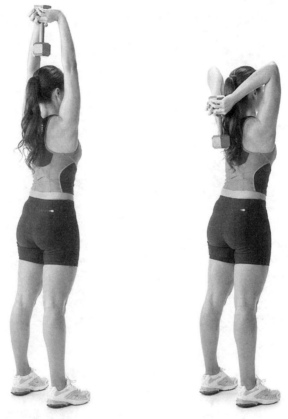

Basic Two-Arm Extension

1. Stand straight, feet shoulder-width apart, holding a dumbbell with both hands.

2. Press the dumbbell over your head and hold it so that your palms are flat against the inside plate—one end of the dumbbell should be pointing up while the other end will be pointing down toward your head.

3. Without moving your upper arms, slowly bend your elbows and lower the dumbbell behind your head as far as possible.

4. Extend the dumbbell back overhead until your arms are straight.

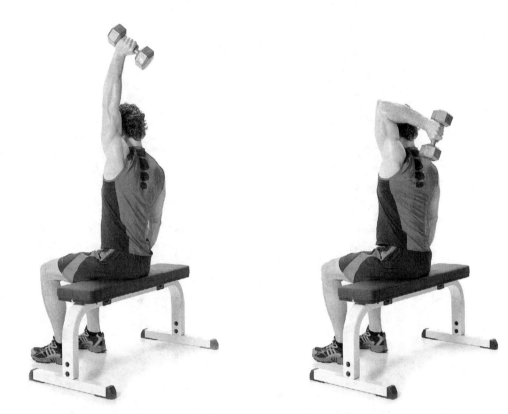

Seated One-Arm Extension

1. Sit on a bench—or sturdy chair—holding a light dumbbell in your left hand.

2. Follow Steps 2–4 of the One-Arm Extension (see page 93).

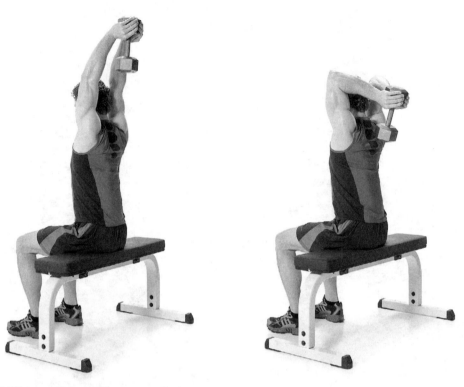

Seated Two-Arm Extension

1. Sit on a bench—or sturdy chair—holding a light dumbbell with both hands.

2. Follow Steps 2–4 of the Two-Arm Extension (see page 94).

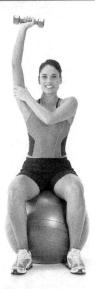 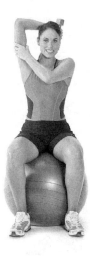

Swiss-Ball One-Arm Extension

1. Sit on a Swiss ball—with your feet wide enough to stay balanced—holding a light dumbbell in your right hand.

2. Follow Steps 2–4 of the One-Arm Extension (see page 93).

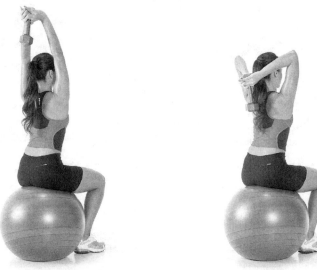

Swiss-Ball Two-Arm Extension

1. Sit on a Swiss ball—with your feet wide enough to stay balanced—holding a light dumbbell with both hands.

2. Follow Steps 2–4 of the Two-Arm Extension (see page 94).

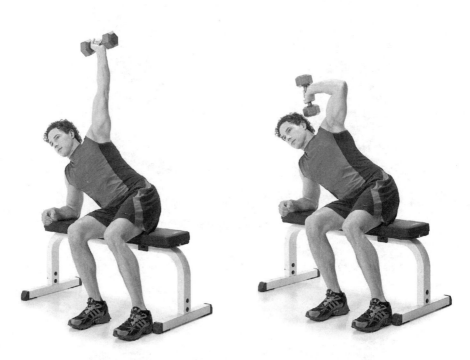

Leaning Unilateral Extension

1. Sit on a bench—or a bed—holding a light dumbbell in your left hand. Place your right hand on the bench, then slide to the right until your body is at a diagonal.

2. Press the dumbbell over your head so that your left arm is straight—palm pointing forward.

3. Without moving your upper arm, slowly bend your left elbow and lower the dumbbell behind your head toward your right ear.

4. Extend the dumbbell back overhead until your left arm is straight and repeat for one set. When you complete the set with your left hand, place the dumbbell in your right hand, lean to the left, and repeat the exercise with your right arm.

Multiply Your Moves! Beginner

There are only *seven* Master Moves when it comes to the triceps extension, but you can still add a few variations to the one-arm versions only.

Dumbbell in Front (creates 4 "new" moves!) Instead of lowering the weight behind your head, try lowering the weight in front of your face. At the start of the exercise, rotate your hand so that your palm faces away from you. This will keep the dumbbell from touching your face as you perform the variation.

Multiply Your Moves! Intermediate

Two Dumbbells (creates 3 "new" moves!) Instead of using two arms (and one dumbbell), try holding a dumbbell in each hand and raise them above you, palms facing in. Slowly lower both dumbbells down behind your head, keeping your upper arms stationary as you go—elbows close—then extend your arms back up.

Multiply Your Moves! Intermediate "Plus"

Two Dumbbells/One Arm at a Time (creates 3 "new" moves!) Instead of lowering both weights, try lowering the weight in your left hand first, keeping your right arm pointing up. Raise the weight back up, then keep your left arm pointing straight up as you lower the weight in your right hand. Take turns using your left arm, then your right, for the entire exercise.

Two Dumbbells/One Up, One Down (creates 3 "new" moves!) Instead of lowering both weights, try lowering the weight in your left hand first, keeping your right arm pointing up. As you raise the weight back up, simultaneously lower the weight in your right hand. Continue the exercise by lowering one weight as you raise the other for the entire set.

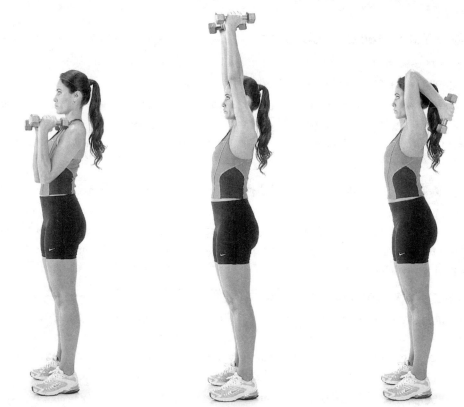

Curl Press Extension

(WORKS YOUR SHOULDERS AND ARMS; CREATES 3 "NEW" MOVES!)

1. Grab a light dumbbell in each hand and let your arms hang down at your sides—you can either stand, sit on a bench, or sit on a Swiss ball.

2. Keeping your palms facing in, curl both weights up to your shoulders.

3. Press the weights over your head—your palms should still be facing each other.

4. Keeping your upper arms stationary, bend your elbows and lower the weights behind your head.

5. Reverse the entire exercise by straightening your arms back overhead, lowering the weights down to your shoulders, then curling them back down to your sides.

>>ADDITIONAL ARM EXERCISES

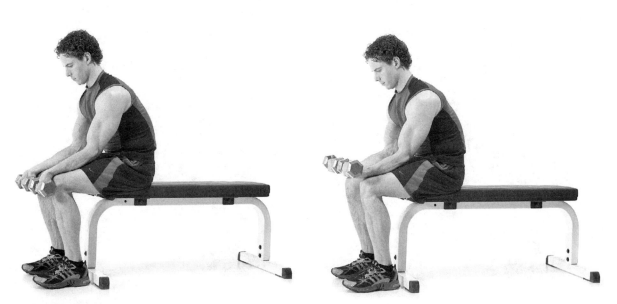

Wrist Curl

(WORKS THE FOREARMS)

1. Sit on a weight bench—or chair—with a light dumbbell in each hand.

2. Lean forward and place your forearms flat on your thighs with your wrists hanging over your kneecaps, palms facing up.

3. Using only your wrists as the hinge for this movement, curl the weights up as far as possible, keeping your forearms against your thighs.

4. Pause, then lower the weights back down as far as you can.

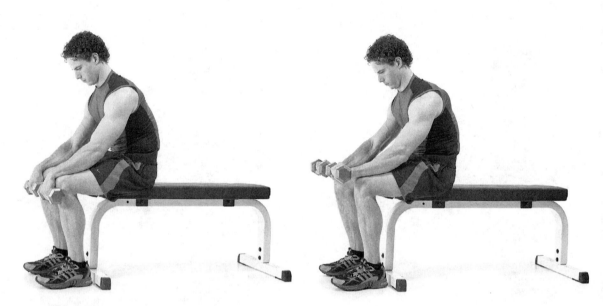

Wrist Extension

(WORKS THE FOREARMS)

1. Sit on a weight bench—or chair—with a light dumbbell in each hand.

2. Lean forward and place your forearms flat on your thighs with your wrists hanging over your kneecaps, palms facing down.

3. Using only your wrists as the hinge for this movement, raise the weights up as far as possible, keeping your forearms against your thighs.

4. Pause, then lower the weights back down.

EXERCISES FOR YOUR
BACK

■ ■ ■

>>BACK ROW

This muscle-shaper works your middle back and latissimus dorsi, as well as your biceps, trapezius, rear shoulders, and brachioradialis. No matter which variation you choose in this section, this exercise is ideal for developing the perfect V-shape back.

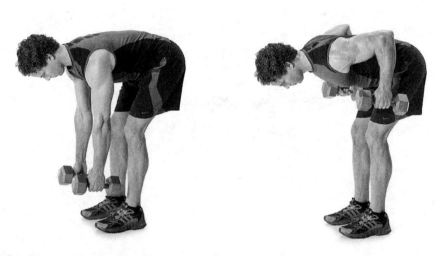

Basic Two-Arm Row

1. Stand with your feet hip-width apart, knees slightly bent and a dumbbell in each hand. Keeping a flat back, bend forward at the waist until your torso is almost parallel to the floor—your arms should extend straight down below you.

2. Turn the weights so that your palms face in.

3. Without moving anything but your arms, slowly pull the dumbbells up close to your body to the sides of your chest.

4. Hold for a second, then lower the weights back down.

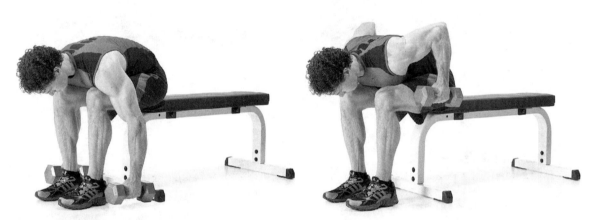

Seated Bent-Over Row

1. Sit on the end of a bench—or a sturdy armless chair—with your knees bent, feet flat on the floor. Place a pair of dumbbells on the floor at your sides. Bend forward at the waist as far as you can until your back is almost parallel to the floor—your chest should touch your legs. Reach down, grab a weight in each hand, and let your arms hang straight down—if they can't, find a chair with a higher seat.

2. Turn the weights so that your palms face in.

3. Without moving anything but your arms, slowly pull the dumbbells up close to your body to the sides of your chest.

4. Hold for a second, then lower the weights back down.

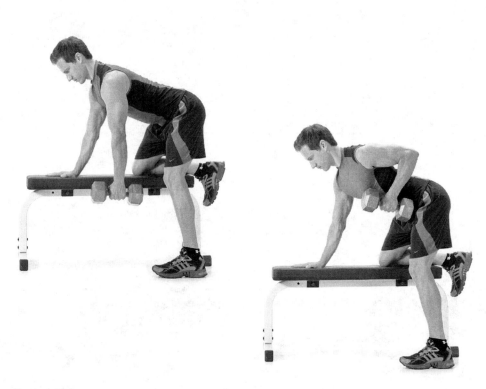

One-Arm Row

Always keep your head, neck, and spine aligned during the exercise. Lifting your head or turning your neck to see the weight can strain your neck muscles. Instead, look down at the bench—or the floor in front of you—as you row.

1. Stand with your right side to an exercise bench. Grab a dumbbell with your left hand, then rest your right hand and right knee on an exercise bench. Lean forward so that your back is almost parallel to the floor and let your left arm hang straight down.

2. Turn the weight so that your palm faces in.

3. Without moving your back, slowly pull the dumbbell up close to your body to the side of your chest.

4. Hold for a second, then lower the weight back down.

5. Finish the set for the required amount of reps, then switch positions and repeat the exercise (this time, placing your left hand and left knee on the bench and holding the weight in your right hand).

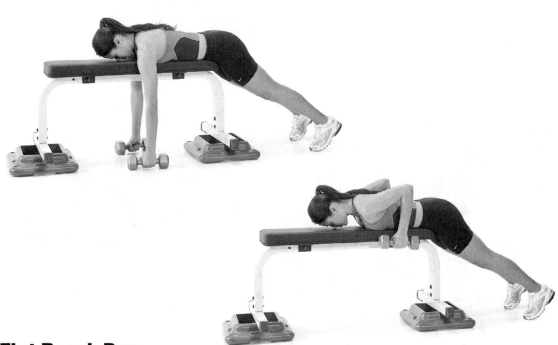

Flat Bench Row

1. Stand in front of one end of a flat bench and lie facedown on it. Shimmy forward until the end of the bench touches your hips—that way, you can bend at the waist and let your knees hang down with your feet touching the floor. Grab a weight in each hand and let your arms hang straight down. (If your arms are too long, try raising the end of the bench by placing an exercise step, a box, etc., underneath it.)

2. Follow Steps 2–4 of the Two-Arm Row (see page 104).

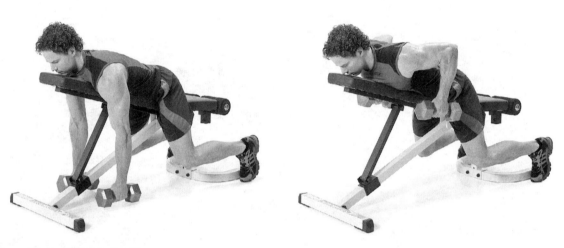

Incline Bench Row

1. Elevate the backrest of an incline bench 1 or 2 notches above a flat position. Grab a dumbbell in each hand, then lie backward on the bench so your chest and abs are flat against the backrest. Your arms should hang straight down.

2. Follow Steps 2–4 of the Two-Arm Row (see page 104).

Multiply Your Moves! Beginner

There are *five* versions of the row in this section, but 112 variations are possible, letting you work your back from every possible angle.

Add a Twist (creates 30 "new" moves!)

If you're starting the exercise the traditional way with your palms facing in—twist the dumbbells as you extend your arms either:

» In so your palms face backward at the end of the move.

» Out so your palms end up facing forward.

If you're starting the exercise with an overhand grip with your palms facing backward—twist the dumbbells out as you row the weight either:

» 90 degrees—so your palms face in at the top.

» 180 degrees—so your palms face forward at the top.

If you're starting the exercise with an underhand grip with your palms facing forward—twist the dumbbells in as you row the weight either:

» 90 degrees—so your palms face in at the top.

» 180 degrees—so your palms face backward at the top.

Regardless of which version you try, reverse the motion as you lower the weights back down so they return to their original position.

Overhand Grip (creates 5 "new" moves!) Twist your wrist(s) so that your palm(s) face backward. Then, keep them in this position as you raise and lower the weight(s).

Underhand Grip (creates 5 "new" moves!) Before you start the exercise, twist your wrist(s) so that your palm(s) face forward. Then, keep them in this position as you raise and lower the weight(s). Use less weight than usual—about 60 to 70 percent less to start.

Multiply Your Moves! Intermediate

Although these two variations don't apply to the One-Arm Row—since that exercise has you working each arm separately—these tweaks apply to the other four variations that have you row both arms together.

One Arm at a Time (creates 4 "new" moves!) Instead of rowing both arms, try rowing one arm at a time, alternating from left to right throughout the exercise.

One Up, One Down (creates 4 "new" moves!) Instead of rowing both arms together, try rowing one arm first, then as you lower it back into the starting position, simultaneously row the opposite arm. Continue the exercise by pulling one weight up as you lower the other weight for the entire set.

Multiply Your Moves! Intermediate "Plus"

Every twist and turn you add to your rows can change the effect of the exercise, bringing in more of your scapular muscles while training your back through a fuller range of motion. Turning the arm also conditions the tiny rotator cuff muscles within your shoulders, making your shoulders less susceptible to overuse injuries from sports, exercise, or everyday activities.

One Arm at a Time + Add a Twist (creates 24 "new" moves!) Choose any of the 24 two-arm versions created by adding any of the six types of twists, but do the exercise one arm at a time.

One Arm at a Time + Overhand Grip (creates 4 "new" moves!) Before you start, twist your wrists so that your palms face backward. Then, keep them in this position as you row the weights up and down one arm at a time.

One Arm at a Time + Underhand Grip (creates 4 "new" moves!) Before you start, twist your wrists so that your palms face forward. Then, keep them in this position as you row the weights up and down one arm at a time.

One Up, One Down + Add a Twist (creates 24 "new" moves!) Choose any of the 24 two-arm versions created by adding any of the twists, but make it more challenging by rowing one weight as you lower the other weight back down.

One Up, One Down + Overhand Grip (creates 4 "new" moves!) Before you start the move, twist your wrists so that your palms face backward. Then, keep them in this position as you row one weight up and lower the other weight down.

One Up, One Down + Underhand Grip (creates 4 "new" moves!) Before you start the move, twist your wrists so that your palms face forward. Then, keep them in this position as you row one weight up and lower the other weight down.

Multiply Your Moves! Advanced

Every single one of the 5 Master Moves and 112 variations in this section has you row the weights up close to your body. Instead, this tweak works more of your upper back and rear shoulders. But for these variations, use about 50 to 60 percent less weight than you usually row to start. If you feel any pain in your shoulders or elbows, stop using this variation immediately.

Wide-Pull Row (creates 117 "new" moves!) Try raising your elbows out to the sides—instead of up and behind you—as you row. Stop once your upper arms are parallel to the floor—your arms should be bent at 90-degree angles with your forearms pointing down to the floor. Lower the weight back down until your arms are once again hanging directly below your shoulders.

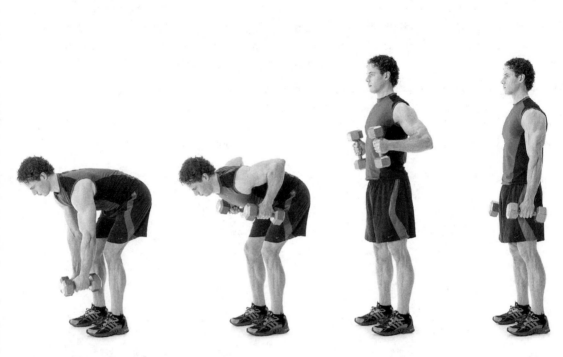

Back Extension Curl Row

(WORKS THE UPPER AND LOWER BACK, PLUS YOUR BICEPS AND FOREARMS)

1. Stand with your feet hip-width apart and a dumbbell in each hand. Bend forward at the waist until your torso is nearly parallel to the floor. Your arms should be extended straight down below you with your palms facing in.

2. Slowly pull the dumbbells up close to your body to the sides of your chest.

3. Keeping the weights tucked along the sides of your body, slowly straighten your back until you're in a standing position.

4. Curl the weights back down, then bend forward again until your torso is almost parallel to the floor—arms extended straight down below you—palms facing in.

5. Repeat Steps 2–4 for the entire set.

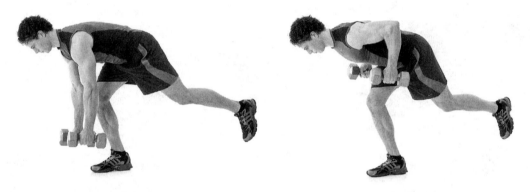

Single-Leg Row

(WORKS THE UPPER AND LOWER BACK, QUADRICEPS, GLUTES, CALVES, AND ABS)

Perform as described, or create 28 "new" moves by adding any of the "Multiply Your Moves!" variations!

1. Stand straight with a light dumbbell in each hand. Raise your left foot off the floor and toward your butt by bending your leg slightly. Slowly bend forward at the waist until your back is almost parallel to the floor, letting your arms hang straight down below you.

2. Follow Steps 2–4 of the Two-Arm Row (see page 104).

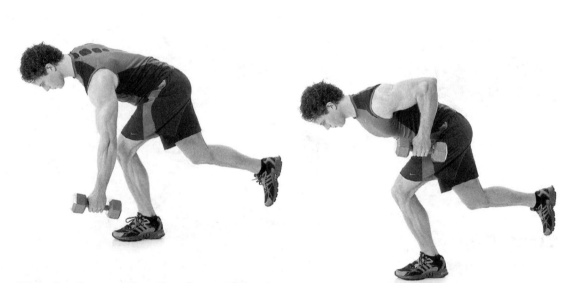

Single-Leg, Single-Arm Row

(WORKS THE BACK, PLUS THE STABILIZING MUSCLES THROUGHOUT EACH LEG)

1. Stand straight with a light dumbbell in your left hand. Raise your right foot off the floor and toward your butt so you're balancing on your left foot. Bend forward until your back is almost parallel to the floor, letting your left arm hang straight down below you, palm facing in.

2. Maintaining your balance, slowly pull the weight up to the side of your chest.

3. Lower the weight back down, finish the set, then repeat the exercise—this time holding the weight in your right hand and balancing on your right foot.

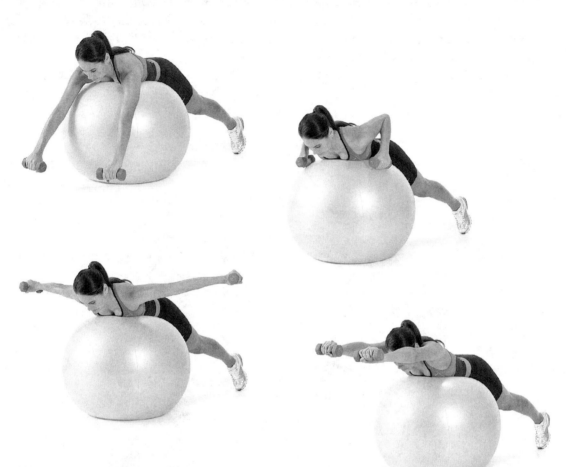

Swiss-Ball Lateral Row

(WORKS THE UPPER BACK, SHOULDERS, AND TRAPEZIUS)

1. Lie facedown on a Swiss ball with a light dumbbell in each hand. Let your arms hang down and position them at a 45-degree angle in front of you with your palms facing backward.

2. Slowly pull the weights up to the sides of your chest, rotating your palms outward as you go, so they end up facing inward at the top.

3. Extend your arms straight out to your sides until they're parallel to the floor, palms facing down.

4. Keeping your arms straight, slowly swing them in front of you, then lower them back down so they're once again at a 45-degree angle.

>>DEADLIFT

This full-body compound exercise works more muscles at the same time than any other single exercise, including your back, legs, gluteal muscles, calves, and abs. Because of its complex nature, there aren't as many variations to choose from, so all of the exercises in this section are Master Moves.

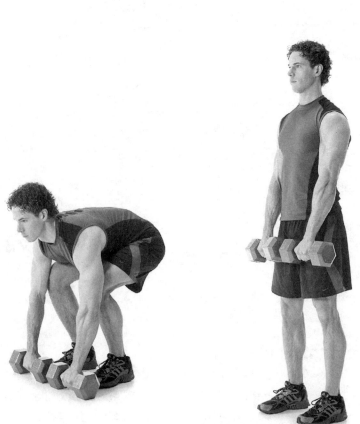

Deadlift

1. Stand straight with your feet hip-width apart and with a pair of heavy dumbbells on the floor in front of your toes. Bend your knees and grab the dumbbells with an overhand grip—palms facing your feet.

2. With your head up and back straight, slowly stand up until your legs are straight, keeping the weights close to your legs as you go.

3. Pause, then reverse the motion and return the weights slowly to the floor.

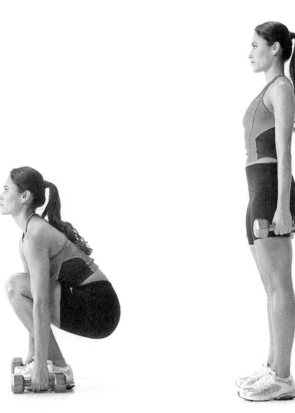

Neutral-Grip Deadlift

1. Stand straight—feet hip-width apart—with a heavy dumbbell placed lengthwise along the outside of each foot. Bend your knees and grab the dumbbells with a neutral grip—palms facing in toward each other.

2. Follow Steps 2–3 of the Deadlift (see opposite page).

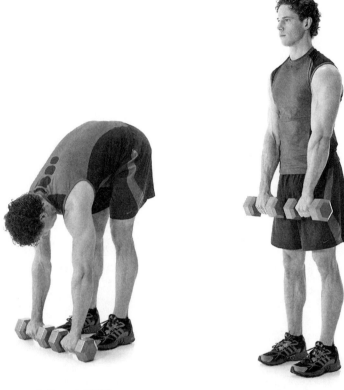

Stiff-Legged Deadlift

This variation doesn't work as many muscles as a regular deadlift, but it does concentrate a lot of effort on your hamstrings and your glutes.

1. Stand straight—feet hip-width apart—with a pair of light dumbbells on the floor about 10 to 12 inches in front of your feet. Keeping your legs straight—knees unlocked—bend forward at the waist and grab the dumbbells with an overhand grip—palms facing your feet.

2. Keeping your back flat and legs straight, slowly lift yourself back up into a standing position, keeping your arms straight as you go.

3. Pause, then reverse the motion and return the weights slowly to the floor.

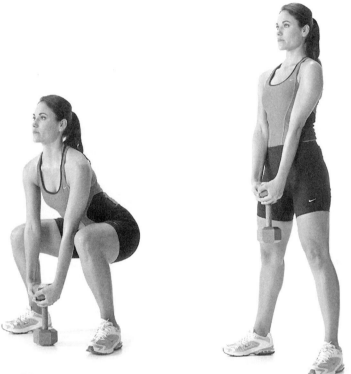

Sumo Deadlift

1. Place a heavy dumbbell on its end, then stand in front of it with your feet wider than shoulder-width apart, toes pointed out to the sides. Bend your knees, reach down, and grab the dumbbell with both hands, wrapping your fingers over the weight plate, palms facing up.

2. With your head up and back straight, slowly stand up until your legs are straight. The weight should hang directly below your waist with your arms extended.

3. Pause, then reverse the motion and return the weight slowly to the floor—keeping the dumbbell resting on its end.

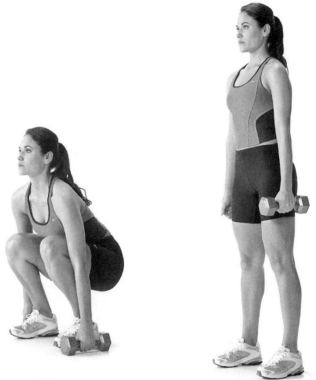

One-Arm Deadlift

1. Stand straight with your feet hip-width apart and a heavy dumbbell on the floor just outside your left foot. Bend your knees and grab the dumbbell with your palm facing in.

2. With your head up and back straight, slowly stand up until your legs are straight, keeping the weight close to your left leg as you go. (Your right arm can hang straight down at your side.)

3. Pause, return the weight slowly to the floor, and finish the set. Then repeat the exercise, this time by holding the weight in your right hand only.

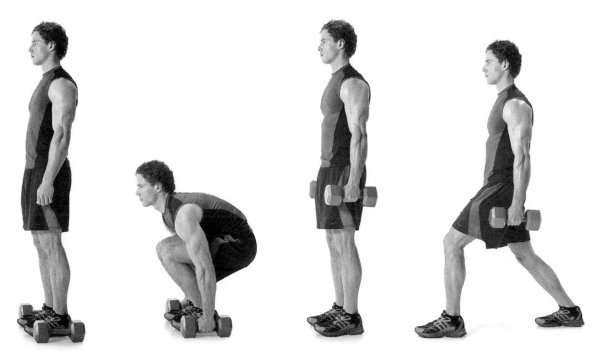

Walking Deadlift

1. Stand straight with your feet hip-width apart and a heavy dumbbell placed lengthwise along the outside of each foot. Bend down and grab the dumbbells with a neutral grip—palms facing in toward each other.

2. With your head up and back straight, slowly stand up until your legs are straight, keeping the weights close to your legs as you go.

3. Once your legs are straight, take one small step forward, leading with your left foot. As soon as your feet are back together again, reverse the motion and lower the weights back to the floor.

4. Repeat the entire exercise leading alternately with your right foot. Continue repeating the exercise, alternating between stepping forward with your left foot first, then your right foot.

Multiply Your Moves! Intermediate "Plus" _____

There are *six* deadlift Master Moves, but there really aren't any ways to safely tweak them. However, on pages 122 and 123, you'll find two "Combine and Conquer" moves to try that can intensify the exercise even further.

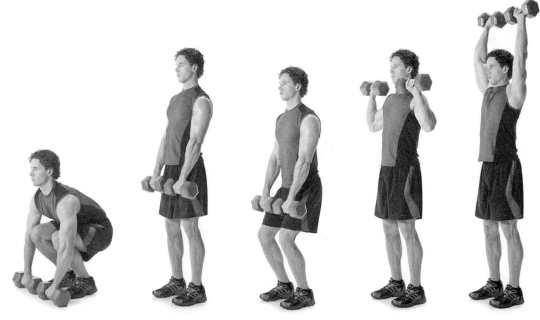

Power Clean and Press

(WORKS THE LEGS, SHOULDERS, TRICEPS, CHEST, BACK, ABDOMINALS, AND GLUTES)

1. Stand with your feet shoulder-width apart and a pair of dumbbells on the floor in front of your feet. Bend your knees and grab both weights with an overhand grip, palms facing your feet.

2. Keeping your back flat, head up, and arms straight, slowly stand up. Your arms should be hanging straight down with the weights resting on your thighs.

3. Next, pushing your weight into the floor for momentum, swing the weights up, bending just your elbows, and catch them on the front of your shoulders. This movement will feel like you're doing a reverse curl, only you'll be using momentum, not your biceps, to swing the weights up into position.

4. Press the weights directly over your head, then reverse the entire process—lower the weights down to your shoulders, curl the weights down until your arms are straight, and finally lower the weights back to the floor.

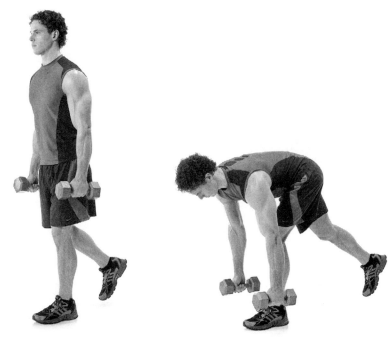

Single-Leg Romanian Deadlift

(WORKS THE BACK, LEGS, AND GLUTES)

1. Stand with a dumbbell in each hand and your arms hanging straight down in front of you—palms facing in.

2. Bend your right leg and raise your right foot behind you so it's a few inches off the floor—you should be balancing on your left foot only.

3. Holding this position, slowly shift your hips backward and bend forward at the waist until your back is almost parallel to the floor.

4. Raise your torso back up into a standing position and repeat for the required amount of reps. Afterward, switch positions—so you're balancing on your right foot only—and repeat the exercise.

>>PULLOVER

This sweeping exercise strengthens the upper back—primarily the lats—as well as the lower chest and triceps.

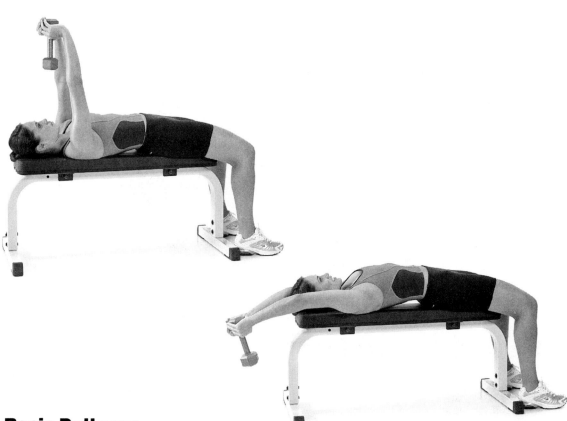

Basic Pullover

1. Lie flat on a bench with your knees bent, feet flat on the floor. Shimmy your body so that your head is right near the end of the bench.

2. Grab a dumbbell and wrap your thumbs and forefingers in a diamond shape around the inside end of the weight, then press it up above your chest with both hands. Your palms should be flat against the inside plate of the dumbbell, palms facing up.

3. With your elbows slightly bent, slowly sweep the weight back behind your head as far as is comfortable—your upper arms should end up alongside your ears.

4. Reverse the motion by sweeping your arms forward—keeping them fixed as you go—until the weight is back over your chest.

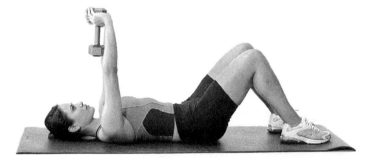

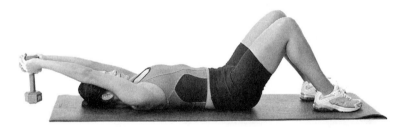

Floor Pullover

1. Lie flat on a carpeted or padded surface with your knees bent, feet flat on the floor.

2. Follow Steps 2–4 of the Basic Pullover (see opposite page), except stop lowering the weight as soon as the end of the dumbbell taps the floor behind you. The range of motion isn't as wide, but it can still strengthen your muscles if you're bench-less.

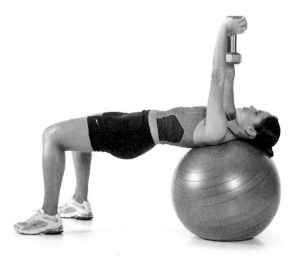

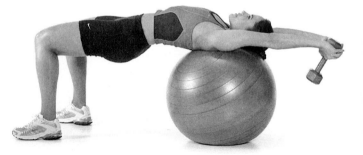

Swiss-Ball Pullover

1. Lie on a Swiss ball—knees bent and feet flat on the floor. Just your head, shoulders, and neck should touch the top of the ball—your lower back shouldn't touch it. Push your hips up so that your torso and thighs form a straight line—parallel to the floor—with your legs bent at 90 degrees.

2. Follow Steps 2–4 of the Basic Pullover (see page 124).

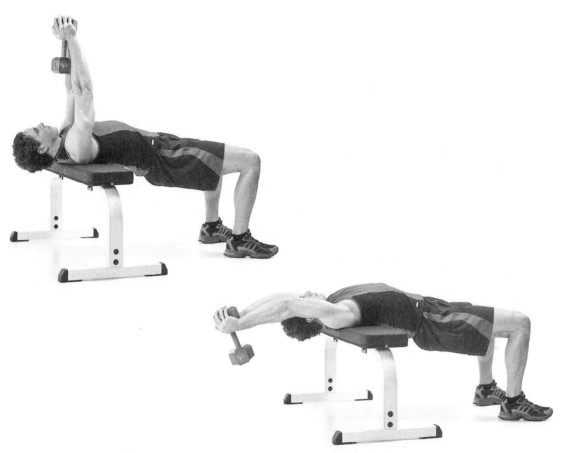

Cross-Bench Pullover

1. Lie perpendicular to a weight bench so that only your shoulders and upper back are resting on it—your head will hang off one side while your body will be on the opposite side. Keeping your knees bent at 90 degrees and your feet flat on the floor, make sure your back is parallel with the floor.

2. Follow Steps 2–4 of the Basic Pullover (see page 124).

Multiply Your Moves! Beginner

There are just *four* Master Move versions of the Pullover to try, but you can make things interesting for your chest muscles by throwing them a few surprise variations like these.

Two Dumbbells (creates 4 "new" moves!) Instead of holding one dumbbell with both hands, try performing the exercise with a dumbbell in each hand. Press the weights together at the top of the exercise—palms facing each other—then keep them together as you lower and raise the weights.

Multiply Your Moves! Intermediate

One Arm at a Time (creates 4 "new" moves!) Instead of lowering both weights behind your head, try lowering the weight in your left hand first, keeping your right arm pointing straight up as you go. Raise the weight back up, then keep your left arm pointing straight up as you lower the weight in your right hand. Alternate using your left and right arms for the entire exercise.

Multiply Your Moves! Intermediate "Plus"

One Up, One Down (creates 4 "new" moves!) Try lowering the weight in your left hand first, keeping your right arm pointing straight up as you go. As you raise the weight back up, simultaneously lower the weight in your right hand. Continue the exercise by alternating for the entire set.

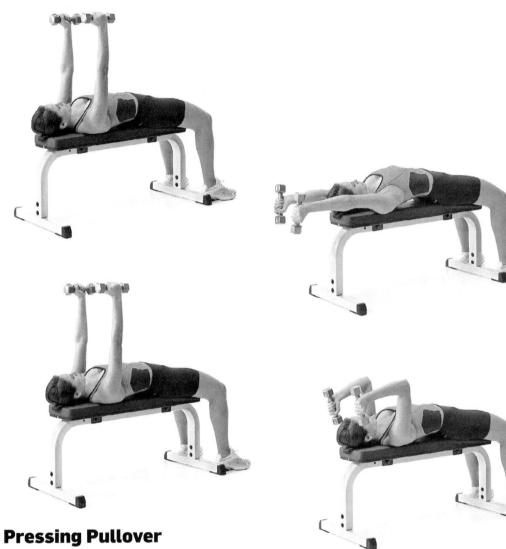

Pressing Pullover

(WORKS THE CHEST, BACK, AND TRICEPS)

In between each pullover, try adding an extension to involve more of your triceps.

1. Perform one repetition of the exercise—sweeping the weight down, then raising it back up.

2. Bend your elbows and lower the weight—or weights—to your head.

3. Press the weights back up.

4. Alternate between doing one pullover and one extension throughout the set.

>>SHRUG

Works the upper back and trapezius muscles—the ones located between your shoulders and your neck.

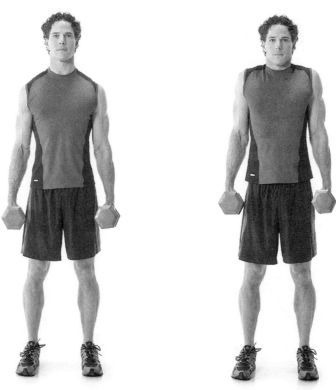

Basic Standing Shrug

1. Stand straight with a heavy dumbbell in each hand, letting your arms hang down along your sides.

2. Turn the weights so that your palms face in toward each other.

3. With your back straight, slowly lift your shoulders up as high as you can—keeping your arms straight as you go.

4. Pause for 1 or 2 seconds, then slowly lower your shoulders down as far as possible.

Note: Do not bend at the elbows as you raise the weights. This only brings your biceps into the exercise to help out. Also, try to keep your shoulders neutral rather than drawing them forward or backward. Rolling your shoulders will only strain your neck muscles. Instead, imagine you're trying to pull your shoulders up to your ears.

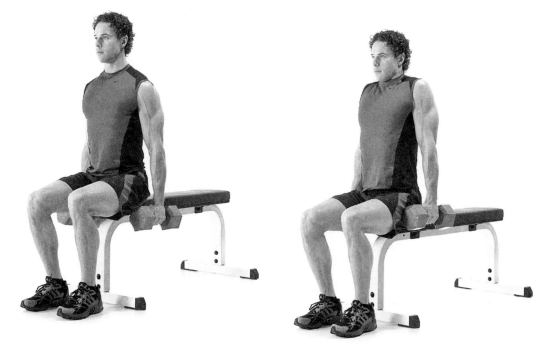

Seated Shrug

1. Sit on the end of a bench—or an armless chair—with a heavy dumbbell in each hand.

2. Follow Steps 2–4 of the Basic Standing Shrug (see opposite page).

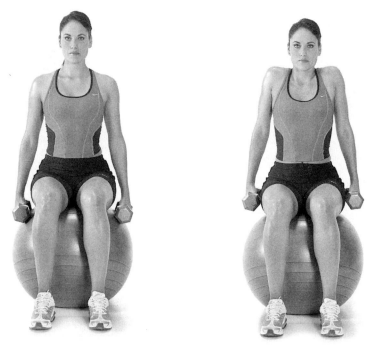

Swiss-Ball Shrug

1. Sit on a Swiss ball with your knees bent and feet flat on the floor, a heavy dumbbell in each hand.

2. Follow Steps 2–4 of the Basic Standing Shrug (see page 130).

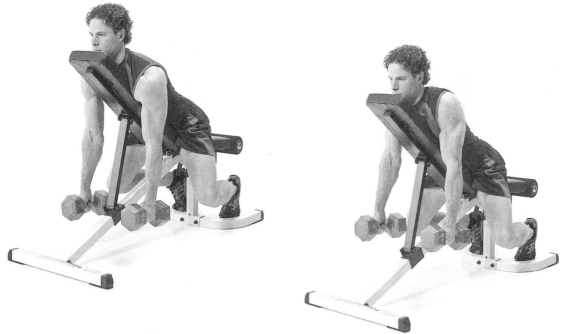

Incline Bench Shrug

1. Set an incline bench at a 30- to 45-degree angle. Grab a heavy dumbbell in each hand. Sit backward on the bench with your chin, chest, and stomach flat against the pad—let your arms hang down below you, palms facing each other.

2. Follow Steps 2–4 of the Basic Standing Shrug (see page 130).

Multiply Your Moves! Beginner

While there are only *four* versions of the Shrug and a handful of interesting ways to alter each version, you can still create 15 exercises when you're looking for something different to try.

In Back/In Front (creates 2 "new" moves!) These two changes place your arms at slightly different angles; however, they can be done only with the Standing Shrug. Instead of letting the weights rest by your sides with your palms facing in, try either:

» Keeping the weights in front of your thighs, palms facing in.

» Placing the weights behind you so they rest on the sides of your butt, palms facing back.

Multiply Your Moves! Intermediate

Reverse Shrug (creates 3 "new" moves!) Instead of letting your arms hang straight down, grab a lighter weight and extend your arms straight up over your head—palms facing each other. Keeping your arms straight, slowly shrug your shoulders up as high as you can, then lower your shoulders back down. *Note:* This can't be done with the incline bench shrug.

One Shoulder at a Time (creates 4 "new" moves!) Instead of raising both shoulders together, raise your left shoulder only. Lower it back down, then raise only your right shoulder. Alternate from left to right throughout the exercise.

Multiply Your Moves! Intermediate "Plus"

Adding the right tweaks can create some interesting possibilities. Here are three you can try when you've tried them all:

One Shoulder at a Time + Reverse Shrug (creates 3 "new" moves!)

One Shoulder at a Time + In Front (creates 1 "new" move!)

One Shoulder at a Time + In Back (creates 1 "new" move!)

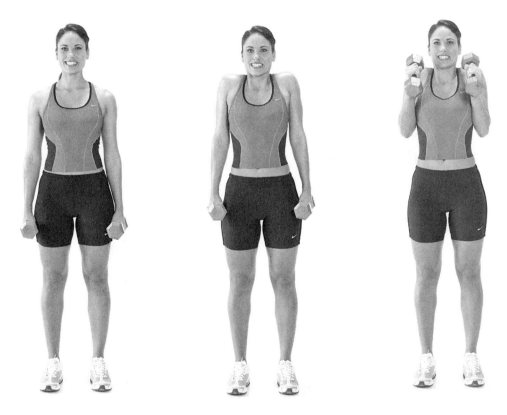

Shrug Curl

(WORKS THE UPPER BACK, SHOULDERS, AND BICEPS

1. Stand straight with a dumbbell in each hand, arms at your sides, palms facing in.

2. Slowly lift your shoulders up as high as you can—keeping your arms straight as you go.

3. Keeping your shoulders raised, slowly curl the weights up to your shoulders, then back down.

4. Finally, lower your shoulders back down.

>>ADDITIONAL BACK EXERCISES

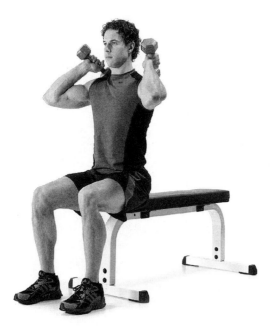

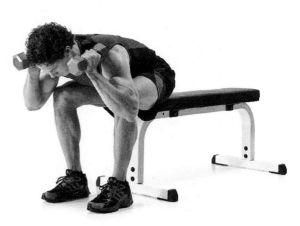

Seated Good Morning

(WORKS THE LOWER BACK)

1. Sit on the end of a bench—or a sturdy armless chair—with a very light dumbbell in each hand. Curl the dumbbells up, rest the ends on your shoulders, and hold them there for the rest of the entire set.

2. Keeping your back flat and the dumbbells held in place, slowly bend forward at the waist and lower your torso as far as you can—keep your head in line with your back as you go. Then, slowly raise your torso back up until you're back in an upright position.

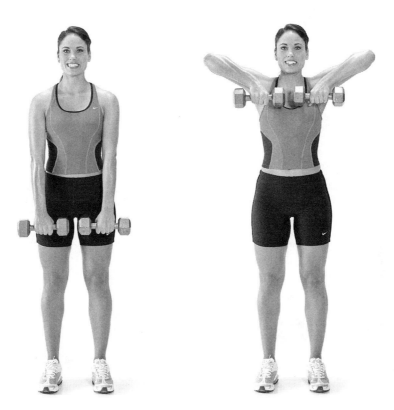

Upright Row

(WORKS THE UPPER BACK, TRAPEZIUS, AND SHOULDERS)

1. Stand straight with your feet hip-width apart, holding a dumbbell in each hand.

2. Position your arms so they hang straight down in front of your body with the weights resting on your thighs—palms facing into your legs.

3. Without moving anything but your arms—your back and legs should remain straight—slowly drag the weights up along the front of your body, leading with your elbows. Keep the dumbbells as close to your body as you can.

4. Raise the weights until they're just below your chin, pause, then lower the weights back down until your arms are straight.

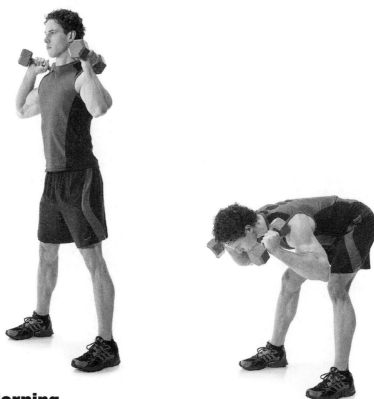

Good Morning

(WORKS THE LOWER BACK)

1. Stand straight with your feet slightly wider than shoulder-width apart and a light dumbbell in each hand. Curl the weights up to your shoulders and rest the ends of the dumbbells on your shoulders—keep them there for the entire set.

2. With your knees unlocked and your back flat, push your hips back and slowly bend over at the waist until your torso is almost parallel to the floor.

3. Raise your torso back up into a standing position.

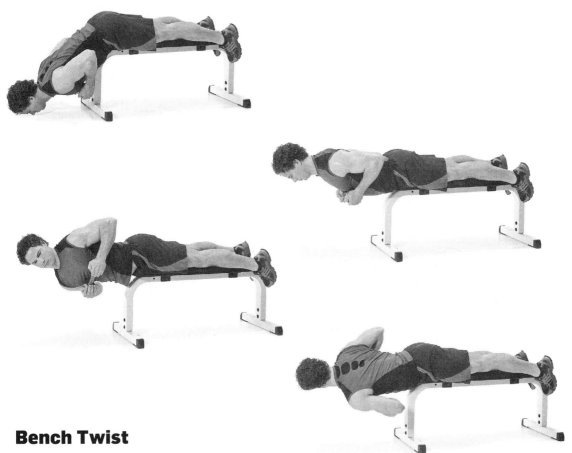

Bench Twist

(WORKS THE LOWER BACK)

1. Lie facedown on an exercise bench and shimmy forward until your torso hangs off the end of the bench—you should be far enough off the bench to be able to bend at the waist. Have a training partner press down on the back of your calves so you stay put—if necessary.

2. Grab a light dumbbell and hold it with both hands to your chest—your elbows will extend to the sides.

3. Bending at the waist, raise your torso up until your body is perfectly straight and parallel to the floor.

4. Slowly turn your torso to your left, then lower yourself back down.

5. Repeat the move—this time, raising up and turning to the right. Alternate from left to right throughout the set.

EXERCISES FOR YOUR
CHEST

>>CHEST FLY

This classic exercise shapes your chest muscles, your front deltoids, and the muscles along your ribs.

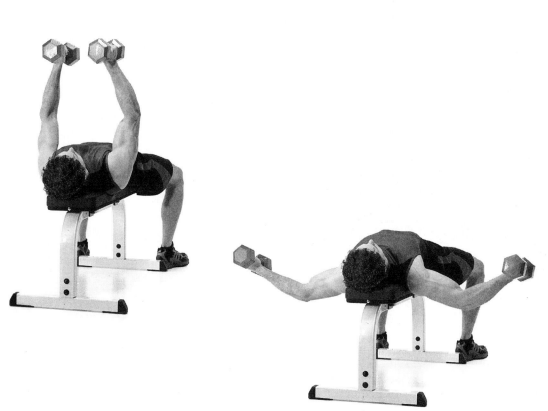

Flat Bench Fly

1. Lie on a flat bench with a dumbbell in each hand. Your knees should be bent with your feet flat on the floor for support.

2. Extend your arms straight up above your chest, palms facing in toward each other with your elbows slightly bent.

3. Keeping your arms fixed in this position, slowly lower your arms out to your sides—in an arclike motion—until the weights are level with your chest.

4. Slowly bring your arms back up (again, in an arclike motion, as if you're wrapping your arms around a big ball) until the weights are once again above your chest.

5. Squeeze your chest muscles for 1 or 2 seconds and repeat.

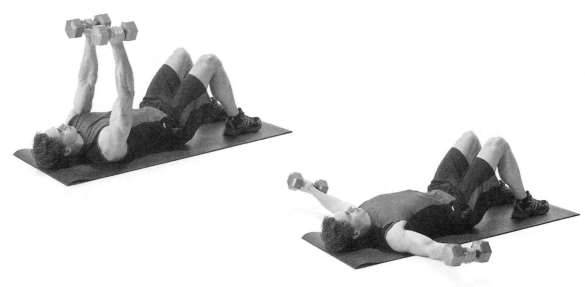

Floor Fly

1. Lie flat on the floor with a dumbbell in each hand. Bend your knees so you can place your feet flat on the floor.

2. Follow Steps 2–5 of the Flat Bench Fly (see page 141).

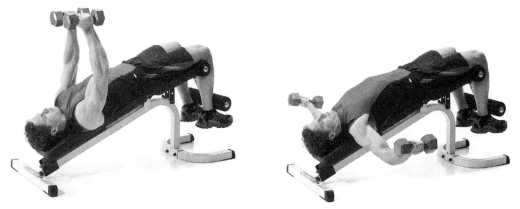

Decline Bench Fly

1. Lie on a decline bench (set at an angle between 30 and 45 degrees below parallel) with a dumbbell in each hand. Secure your feet at the high end of the bench for support.

2. Follow Steps 2–5 of the Flat Bench Fly (see page 141).

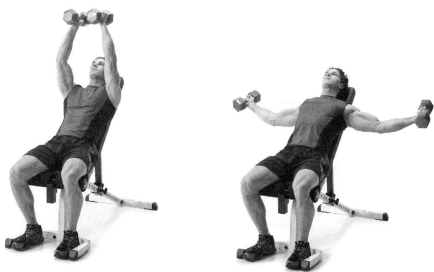

Incline Bench Fly

1. Lie on an incline bench with a dumbbell in each hand. Your knees should be bent with your feet flat on the floor for support.

2. Follow Steps 2–5 of the Flat Bench Fly (see page 141).

Multiply Your Moves! Intermediate "Plus"—*Continued*

Add a Twist + One Arm at a Time (creates 12 "new" moves!) Try any of the 12 versions created by adding either twist, but make it more of a challenge by lowering the weight in one hand while keeping the other arm pointed up above you.

Overhand Grip + Feet Raised (creates 3 "new" moves!) Before you start, twist your wrists so your palms face forward and raise your feet up on the bench. Keep them in this position as you perform the exercise.

Add a Twist + Feet Raised (creates 6 "new" moves!) Try any of the 12 versions created by adding either twist, but make it more of a challenge by placing your feet up on the bench.

Multiply Your Moves! Advanced

These changes are only for those exercisers who have paid their dues, so try them only if you're experienced. If you feel any pain or discomfort in your joints, stop immediately.

Elbows Locked (creates 42 "new" moves!) Instead of having a slight bend in your arms as you do the exercise, use a pair of dumbbells that are between 60 and 70 percent less weight than you normally use and try the exercise with your arms straight, elbows locked. *Note:* Because this move requires more balance, don't try it with any of the "Feet Raised" variations.

Loose Hands (creates 60 "new" moves!) Every version of the chest fly demands that you keep a firm grip on both dumbbells, but this tweak can strengthen your forearms while placing the emphasis of the exercises on your chest muscles when you are in the "down" position of the move. To do it, start with the weights above you, then bring them out to your sides as usual.

Once your arms are out to your sides, open your hands *slightly* until you feel your arms working just to keep the dumbbells balanced in your palms. Hold this pose for 1 or 2 seconds, then slowly draw your arms back up as you simultaneously tighten your grip on each dumbbell—you should have a firm grip on the weights when they are about halfway from being back above you.

Unbalanced Grip (creates 324 "new" moves!) Every exercise in this section—including all 156 variations up until now—has you holding the dumbbells in the center of the handle. Instead, try sliding your hands either all the way to the left or the right of the handle. Look at your hands and they will be in one of two positions:

» The thumb side of your hand(s) will be pressed against the inside plate of the dumbbell(s).

» The pinky side of your hand(s) will be pressed against the inside plate of the dumbbell(s).

The weights will feel off-center in your hands, no matter which way you choose to slide your hands. This unevenness forces your chest to work twice as hard to help balance the weights as you go.

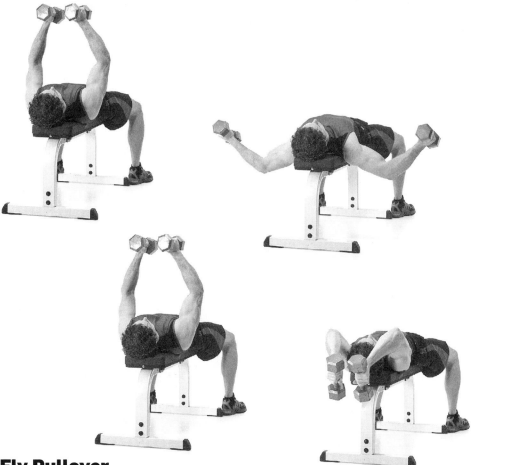

Fly Pullover

(WORKS THE CHEST, TRICEPS, AND UPPER BACK)

You can also do this exercise using three different variations from the "Multiply Your Moves!" section (Overhand Grip, Add a Twist, and Feet Raised) for a total of at least 24 more possible variations.

1. Perform Steps 1–5 of the Chest Fly (see page 141), lowering and raising your arms for one rep. Your arms should end up extended straight above your chest, palms facing in toward each other, elbows slightly bent.

2. Keeping your arms fixed in this position, slowly sweep your arms down and lower both weights below your head, keeping your arms straight—elbows unlocked—as you go.

3. Slowly pull your arms back into the starting position—directly over your chest, arms out to your sides—in an arclike motion, until the weights are level with your chest.

≫CHEST PRESS

Considered to be the most effective exercise for developing your chest muscles, this powerful move also works your shoulders and triceps at the same time.

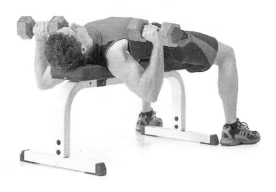
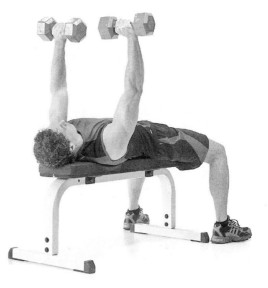

Basic Chest Press

1. Lie flat on an exercise bench—knees bent and feet flat on the floor—holding a dumbbell in each hand. Position the weights along the sides of your chest, elbows aimed at the floor.

2. Turn the weights so that your palms face forward.

3. Keeping your back flat on the bench, slowly press the weights up until your arms are fully extended above your chest, elbows unlocked.

4. Slowly lower the weights back down along the sides of your chest and repeat.

Note: Rounding your back—as many exercisers tend to do—not only helps you cheat the weight up by using additional muscles but also can strain your lower back if you're not careful. So remember to keep your back and butt flat on the bench. If you have to arch your back, you're using dumbbells that are too heavy for you.

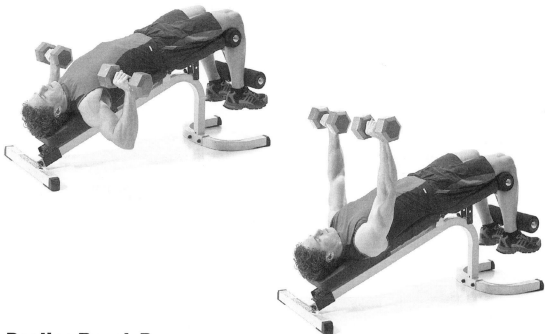

Decline Bench Press

You may not realize it, but the angle of a decline bench decreases the distance you have to push the weight up. Because of this, you'll discover your chest muscles are much stronger lying in this position, so choose dumbbells that are between 10 and 20 percent heavier than you use when doing a standard Chest Press.

1. Lie on a decline bench (set at an angle between 30 and 45 degrees below parallel) and secure your feet at the high end of the bench for support. Grab a dumbbell in each hand and position the weights along the sides of your chest, elbows aimed at the floor.

2. Follow Steps 2–4 of the Basic Chest Press (see opposite page).

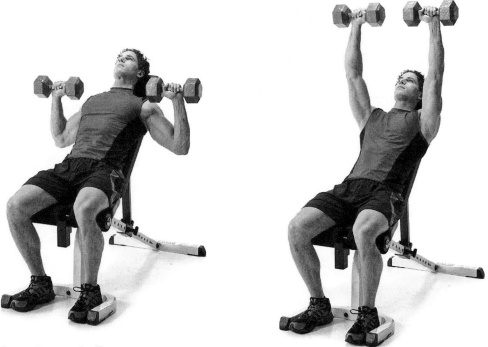

Incline Bench Press

Just like the Decline Bench Press, performing the chest press from this position stresses your chest from a different angle, incorporating more muscle fibers along the upper portions of your chest.

1. Lie flat on an incline bench with your knees bent and feet flat on the floor. Grab a dumbbell in each hand and position the weights along the sides of your chest, elbows aimed at the floor.

2. Follow Steps 2–4 of the Basic Chest Press (see page 148).

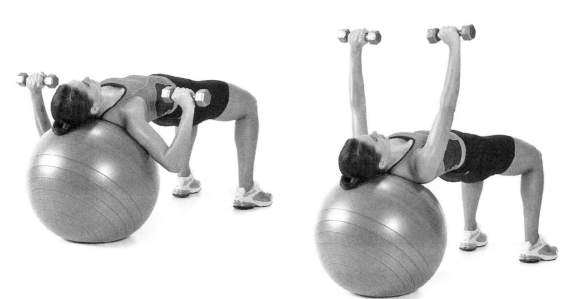

Swiss-Ball Chest Press

Balancing on a Swiss ball takes a lot of concentration, but lying across it for this variation trains your body to maintain its balance as you press, teaching your entire body to work more effectively with your chest muscles.

1. Lie faceup on a Swiss ball—knees bent and feet flat on the floor. Just your head, shoulders, and neck should touch the top of the ball—your lower back should be out and away from it. Push your hips up so that your torso and thighs form a straight line—parallel to the floor—with your legs bent at 90 degrees.

2. Position the weights along the sides of your chest, elbows aimed at the floor.

3. Follow Steps 2–4 of the Basic Chest Press (see page 148).

Multiply Your Moves! Intermediate

Instead of pressing both weights at the same time, these alterations make the move much more difficult to do, forcing other muscles within your body—especially your core muscles—to help stabilize your body as you do it.

One Arm at a Time (creates 5 "new" moves!) Instead of pressing both weights up and down simultaneously, try pressing the weight in your left hand first. Lower the weight back down, then repeat the exercise, this time pressing the weight in your right hand. Alternate from left to right throughout the exercise.

One Up, One Down (creates 5 "new" moves!) Instead of pressing both weights together, try pressing the weight in your left hand first without moving your right arm. As you lower the weight in your left hand, simultaneously press the weight in your right hand. Continue the exercise by pressing one weight as you lower the other for the entire set.

Multiply Your Moves! Intermediate "Plus"

There are a lot of variations to choose from after you've mastered the basics. Here are just a handful that will keep your chest guessing.

Close Grip (creates 5 "new" moves!) Instead of bringing the weights down to your shoulders when lowering them, bring the weights together at the top of the move and keep them close to each other as you lower them. This brings more of your triceps into the exercise than usual.

One Arm at a Time + Neutral Grip (creates 5 "new" moves!) Before you start, twist your wrists in so that your palms face each other. Then, keep them in this position as you press and lower the weights one arm at a time.

One Arm at a Time + Reverse Grip (creates 5 "new" moves!) Before you start, twist your wrists in so that your palms face your shoulders. Then, keep them in this position as you press and lower the weights one arm at a time.

One Arm at a Time + Add a Twist (creates 30 "new" moves!) Try any of the 30 versions created by adding any of the six types of twists, but up the intensity by doing the exercise one arm at a time.

One Up, One Down + Neutral Grip (creates 5 "new" moves!) Before you start, twist your wrists in so that your palms face each other. Then, keep them in this position as you press one weight as you lower the other.

One Up, One Down + Reverse Grip (creates 5 "new" moves!) Before you start, twist your wrists in so that your palms face your shoulders. Then, keep them in this position as you press one weight as you lower the other.

One Up, One Down + Add a Twist (creates 30 "new" moves!) Try any of the 30 versions created by adding any of the six types of twists, but make it more of a challenge by pressing the weight in one hand as you lower the weight in the other.

Multiply Your Moves! Advanced

Two of these three tweaks work with all 140 versions of the chest press in this section, but they intensify all of them by requiring extreme balance and concentration. If you feel too shaky using them, wait until you've had more experience using the other options in this section.

Feet Raised (creates 56 "new" moves!) Instead of keeping your feet flat on the floor, raise them and either place them on the end of the bench or just keep them suspended off the floor as you do the exercise.

Uneven Weights (creates 140 "new" moves!) Instead of holding a pair of dumbbells of equal weight, pick one dumbbell that's the weight you typically use and pick another that's either slightly heavier or lighter (a difference of 2.5 to 5 pounds is usually enough). Perform any variation as described for one set, then switch the heavier weight to the opposite hand for the second set. If a routine requires you to perform an odd amount of sets (three, five, etc.), then do half the repetitions on your last set, then switch the weights in your hands before finishing the final set.

Unbalanced Grip (creates 672 "new" moves!) Every exercise in this section—including all variations up until now—has you holding the dumbbells in the center of the handle. Instead, try sliding your hands either all the way to the left or the right of the handle. Look at your hands and they will be in one of two positions:

» The thumb side of your hand(s) will be pressed against the inside plate of the dumbbell(s).

» The pinky side of your hand(s) will be pressed against the inside plate of the dumbbell(s).

The weights will feel off-center in your hands, no matter which way you choose to slide your hands. This unevenness forces your chest to work twice as hard to help balance the weights as you go.

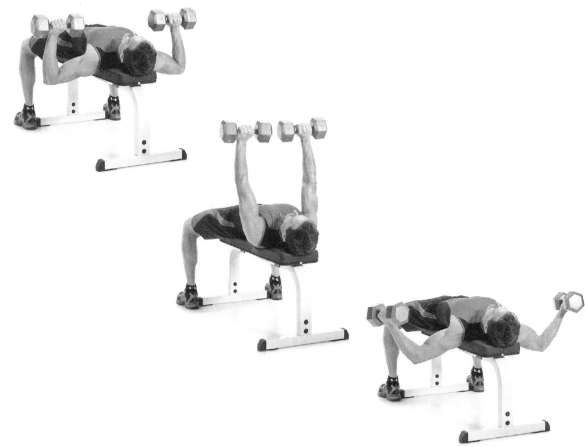

Fly Press

(WORKS THE CHEST, SHOULDERS, AND TRICEPS)

1. Lie flat on an exercise bench, holding a dumbbell in each hand. Position the weights along the sides of your chest, palms facing forward.

2. Slowly press the weights up until your arms are fully extended above your chest, elbows unlocked.

3. Keeping your arms straight, slowly lower your arms out to your sides—in an arclike motion—until the weights are level with your chest. As you lower your arms, rotate the weights out so that your palms end face up.

4. Slowly bring your arms back up until the weights are once again above you, then lower the weights back down to your chest, rotating the weights in so that your palms once again face forward.

≫ADDITIONAL CHEST EXERCISES

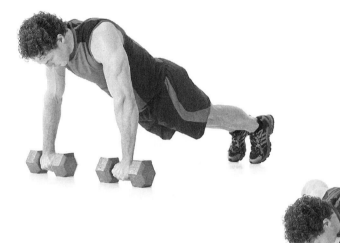

Pushup

(WORKS THE CHEST, SHOULDERS, AND TRICEPS)

1. Kneel down on the floor with two dumbbells on the floor in front of you spaced shoulder-width apart. Grab the dumbbells with an overhand grip and get into a pushup position—your arms should be straight, elbows unlocked, and your legs extended behind you, feet together.

2. Keeping your back straight, bend your elbows and lower your body to the floor.

3. Push yourself back up until your arms are straight, elbows unlocked.

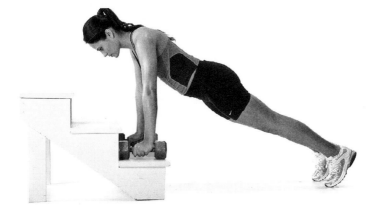

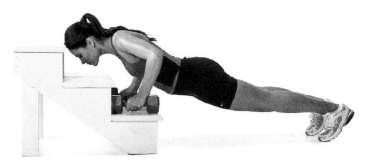

Step Decline Pushup

(WORKS THE CHEST, SHOULDERS, AND TRICEPS)

Follow the same instructions as the Pushup (see page 157), except instead of placing the dumbbells on the floor, place them up on a step or a stair. Your upper body will be elevated as you perform the exercise.

Note: This exercise isn't actually more difficult than doing the exercise on the floor. However, it angles your arms in a position that mimics the Decline Chest Press. This tweak not only redirects some of the stress onto different muscle fibers within your chest, but it also lets you perform even more pushups than usual—perfect for improving muscular endurance.

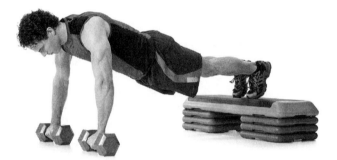

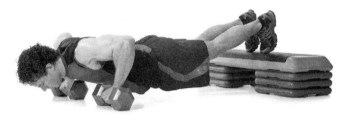

Step Incline Pushup

(WORKS THE CHEST, SHOULDERS, AND TRICEPS)

Follow the same instructions as the Pushup (see page 157), except instead of keeping your feet on the floor, place them up on a step or stair. Your legs will be elevated as you perform the exercise.

Note: This exercise is more difficult than doing the exercise on the floor. It angles your arms in a position that mimics the Incline Chest Press, an angle that makes it harder to perform the move—ideal for seasoned exercisers who find traditional pushups to be too easy to do.

Multiply Your Moves!

These variations apply to all types of pushups, making them even more intense for your upper body. There are no beginner variations.

Multiply Your Moves! Intermediate

Close Grip (creates 3 "new" moves!) Instead of spacing the dumbbells shoulder-width apart, bring them in closer so you start the exercise with the dumbbells 4 to 6 inches from each other.

Multiply Your Moves! Intermediate "Plus"

One Leg (creates 3 "new" moves!) Instead of keeping both feet on the floor (or step), raise one foot an inch or two off the floor and keep it suspended as you perform the exercise. Switch feet when repeating the exercise for a second set.

Row Each Dumbbell (creates 3 "new" moves!) In between each pushup, place your body weight on your right hand and row the dumbbell in your left hand up to the side of your chest. Put the weight back down, then place your body weight on your left hand and row the weight in your right hand up to the side of your chest.

Uneven Hands (creates 3 "new" moves!) Instead of holding both dumbbells, hold a dumbbell with one hand and place the other hand flat on the floor—your body will be uneven for the entire set. Switch hands when repeating the exercise for a second set.

Multiply Your Moves! Advanced

Raise Each Dumbbell (creates 3 "new" moves!) As you push yourself up, rotate your body to the left, lift the dumbbell in your left hand off the floor, and extend it straight up toward the ceiling (your body will look like a T). Twist back down, place the dumbbell back on the floor, then do another pushup. As you push yourself up, this time rotate to the right and extend the dumbbell in your right hand up to the ceiling. Keep alternating from left to right throughout the set.

EXERCISES FOR YOUR
LEGS

>>CALF RAISE

This lower-leg exercise not only shapes the calf muscles but also helps make them stronger so you can handle more weight in many major leg-building exercises, including the squat and the lunge.

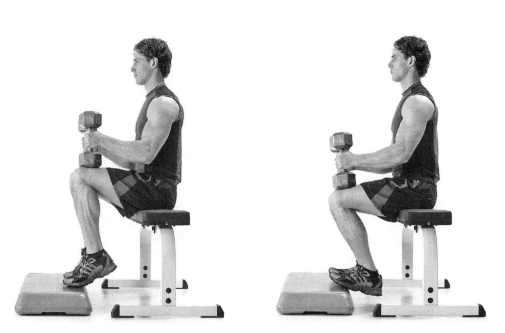

Seated Calf Raise

1. Sit on the edge of a bench—or chair—and place a small block, step, etc.. by your feet. (An exercise step will work as will a piece of wood. You can even try setting the bench in front of a staircase.)

2. Place just the balls of your feet on the step so that your heels hang off the edge.

3. Grab a dumbbell in each hand and place the ends of the weights just above your knees (on the lowest part of your thighs).

4. Holding them in place, raise your heels as high as you can by pushing down with your toes.

5. Pause for 1 or 2 seconds, then slowly lower your heels down as far as you can. (*Note:* To ensure the greatest range of motion—and the best results—your heels should never be able to touch the floor. If they do, then the step you're using is too low, so adjust accordingly.)

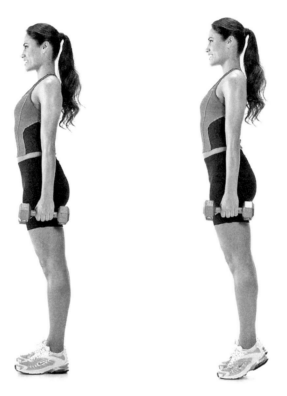

Two-Leg Calf Raise

1. Stand straight with your feet hip-width apart and a heavy dumbbell in each hand, arms by your sides.

2. Keeping your back straight, slowly rise up on the toes of both feet, raising your heels as high as you can.

3. Pause at the top, then slowly lower your heels back down.

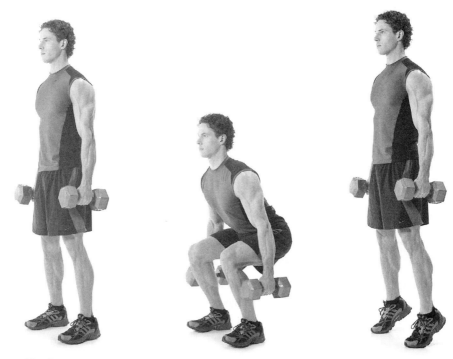

Squat Raise

(WORKS YOUR LEGS, GLUTES, AND CALVES)

1. Stand straight holding a dumbbell in each hand—feet hip-width apart—with your arms at your sides, palms facing in.

2. Slowly squat down until your thighs are parallel to the floor, then stand back up. But instead of pressing through your heels, try pressing through your toes as you go.

3. Once your legs are straight, raise your heels off the floor as high as possible.

4. Hold for a second, then lower your feet back to the floor.

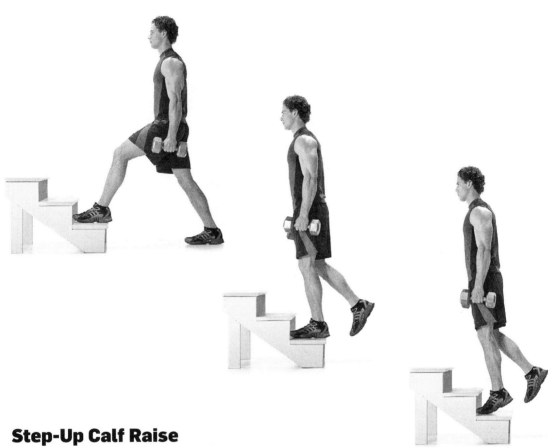

Step-Up Calf Raise

(WORKS THE LEGS, GLUTES, AND CALVES)

1. Stand in front of a step with a light dumbbell in both hands and place your left foot flat on the step.

2. Push off with your right foot, straighten your left leg, and rise up onto the step, balancing on your left foot only.

3. Immediately raise your left heel as high as you can, then reverse the motion by lowering yourself back down, placing your right foot back on the floor so you end up back in the starting position.

4. Finish the set, then switch legs—this time, placing your right foot on the step.

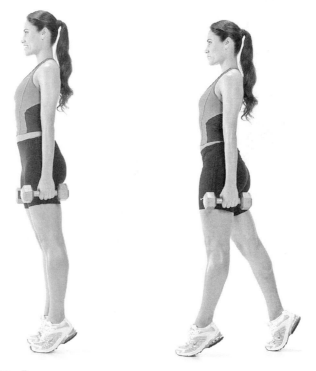

Walking Calf Raise

(WORKS THE LEGS, CALVES, AND FOREARMS)

1. Stand straight with a heavy dumbbell in each hand, arms down at your sides.

2. Rise up on the balls of your feet, then walk forward—keeping your heels off the floor as you go—for as many steps as you can.

>>LUNGE

Not only does this stability-challenging leg exercise train everything from the waist down, including your hamstrings, quadriceps, glutes, and calves, but it also teaches your body better balance.

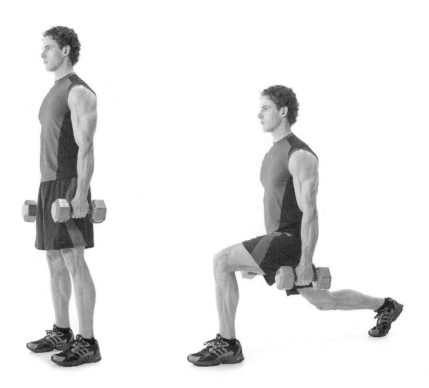

Lunge

1. Stand straight with your feet about 6 inches apart and a dumbbell in each hand.

2. Your arms should hang straight down from your sides, palms facing in.

3. Take a big step forward with your left foot and lower your body until your left thigh is almost parallel to the floor. Your right leg should be extended behind you with only the ball of your right foot on the floor.

4. Reverse the motion by pressing yourself back up into a standing position, then perform the exercise again, this time by taking a big step forward with your right foot. Alternate from left to right throughout the set.

Note: Don't lunge so far forward that your knee extends past your foot. This puts stress around the kneecap and can lead to injury. Your lead leg should be bent at a 90-degree angle in the down position.

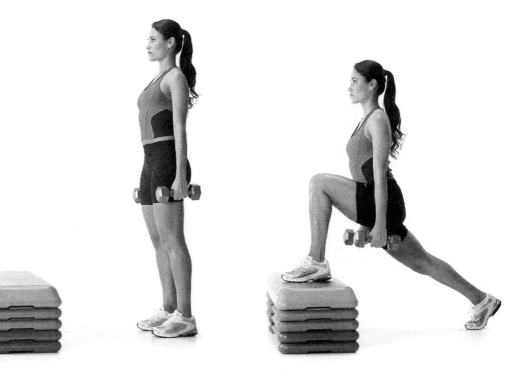

Step Lunge

1. Stand about 2 to 3 feet behind an exercise step—or staircase—with your feet about 6 inches apart and a dumbbell in each hand (palms facing in).

2. With your left foot, step forward and place your entire foot on the step—or the first stair. Slowly lunge forward until your left thigh is parallel to the floor.

3. Reverse the motion by pushing off the step so you're back in a standing position. Perform the exercise again, this time by stepping forward with your right foot. Alternate from left to right throughout the set.

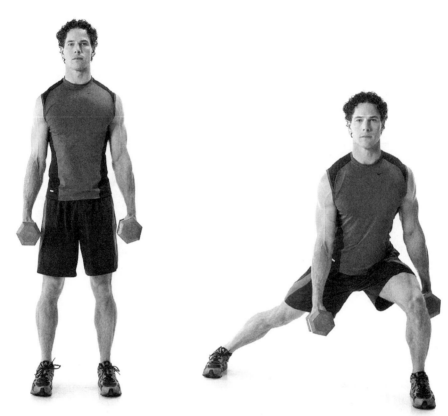

Side Lunge

1. Stand straight with a dumbbell in each hand, arms down at your sides, palms facing in.

2. Keeping your torso facing forward, take a wide step out to the left with your left foot, keeping your toes pointed forward.

3. Bend your left knee until your left thigh is almost parallel to the floor—your right leg will be straight and at an angle.

4. Push yourself back up, then repeat the exercise by taking a wide step out to the right with your right foot. Alternate from left to right throughout the set.

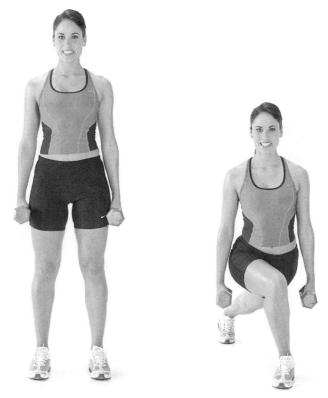

Sidestep Lunge

1. Stand straight with a dumbbell in each hand—arms at your sides—and your feet shoulder-width apart.

2. Take a step back with your left leg, placing your left foot across and a few feet behind your right foot as you simultaneously bend your right knee. Don't rotate your torso as you lunge. Stop once your right thigh is almost parallel to the floor.

3. Push yourself back into a standing position and repeat the exercise, this time stepping back with your right foot and planting it across and behind your left foot.

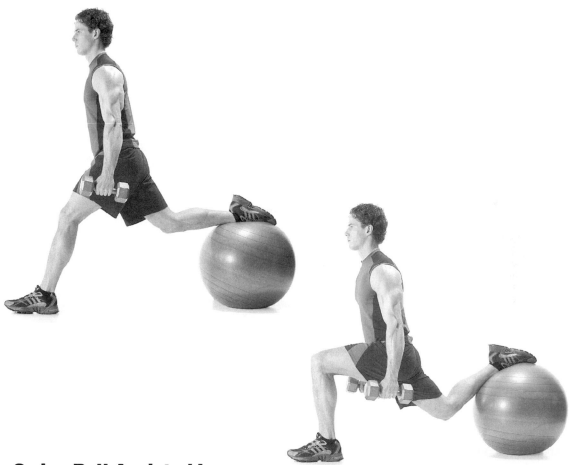

Swiss-Ball Assisted Lunge

1. Stand straight with a dumbbell in each hand and your back about 2 to 3 feet away from a Swiss ball. Extend your right foot back behind you and rest the top of your foot on the ball.

2. Follow Steps 2–3 of the Assisted Lunge (see page 172).

Multiply Your Moves! Beginner

There are *9* lunge Master Moves, but just a handful of variations that you can try. But don't worry, you'll learn how to double, triple, and quadruple every single move in this book—including these 10 Master Moves—in a later chapter.

Weights on Shoulders (creates 9 "new" moves!) Instead of letting your arms hang down at your sides, curl the weights up and rest the ends of the dumbbells on the front of your shoulders.

Multiply Your Moves! Intermediate

Arms Overhead (creates 9 "new" moves!) Instead of letting your arms hang down at your sides, use lighter weights than usual and press them over your head. Then, hold them there for the entire exercise.

Multiply Your Moves! Intermediate "Plus"

One Arm Overhead (creates 9 "new" moves!) Instead of letting your arms hang down at your sides, use a *single* lighter dumbbell than usual and press it over your head with your right arm. Then, hold it above your head as you lunge forward with your *left* leg only. After you complete a set with your left leg, switch the weight to your left hand, extend it overhead, and repeat the exercise with your right leg.

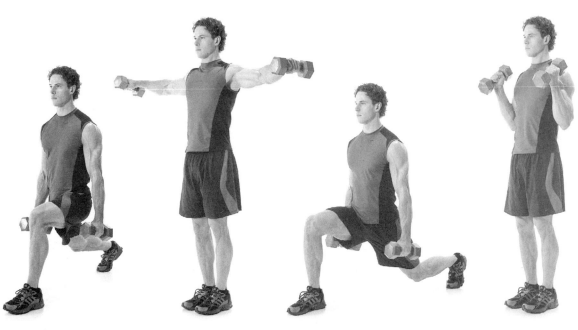

Full-Body Lunge

(WORKS THE LEGS, BACK, SHOULDERS, BICEPS, FOREARMS, GLUTES, AND CALVES)

1. Follow Steps 1–4 of the Lunge (see page 169), stepping forward with your left leg, then step back into a standing position.

2. Next, slowly raise your arms from your sides until they're parallel to the floor, then lower the weights back down to your sides.

3. Repeat Steps 1–4 of the Lunge again, this time stepping forward with your right leg, then step back into a standing position.

4. Curl the weights up to your shoulders, then slowly lower the weights back down to your sides.

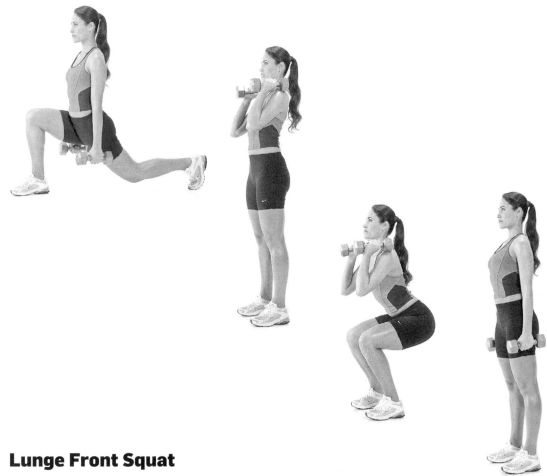

Lunge Front Squat

(WORKS THE ENTIRE LOWER BODY AND THE BICEPS)

1. Follow Steps 1–4 of the Lunge (see page 169), stepping forward first with your left leg, and then with your right leg.

2. Before repeating the two-part cycle, immediately curl the weights up and rest the ends of the dumbbells on your shoulders.

3. Bend *both* legs and squat down until your thighs are parallel to the floor, then stand back up.

4. Curl the weights back down to your sides.

5. Keep alternating between two lunges, one curl, and one squat throughout the exercise.

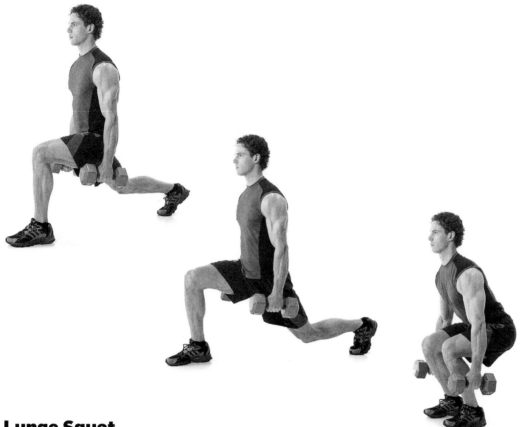

Lunge Squat

(WORKS THE ENTIRE LOWER BODY)

1. Follow Steps 1–4 of the Lunge (see page 169), stepping forward first with your left leg, and then with your right leg.

2. Before repeating the two-part cycle, immediately bend *both* legs and squat down until your thighs are parallel to the floor, then stand back up.

3. Keep alternating between two lunges and one squat throughout the exercise.

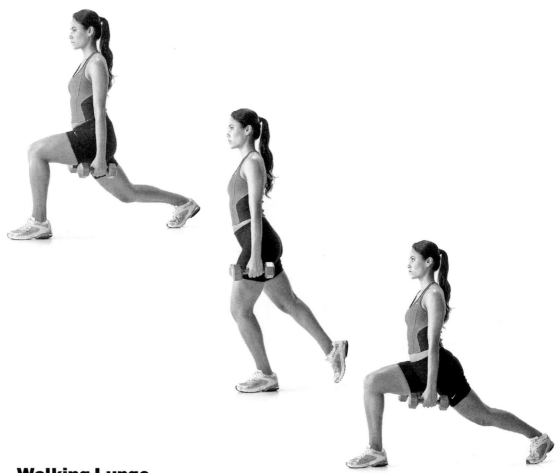

Walking Lunge

(WORKS THE LEGS AND GLUTES)

Follow Steps 1–3 of the Lunge (see page 169), but instead of pushing yourself back into a standing position, put all your weight on your lead leg, then stand back up, bringing your back leg forward so you've traveled one full stride. Keep lunging forward—alternating between your left and right legs—across the room.

»SQUAT

This classic exercise targets all of the muscles within your lower body—including your quadriceps, hamstrings, and calf muscles.

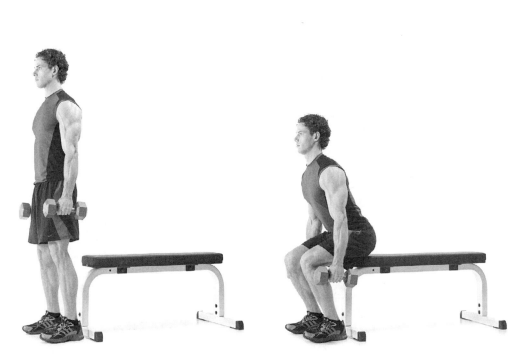

Bench Squat

1. Stand with your back to the end of a weight bench—or chair—holding a dumbbell in each hand. Your feet should be hip-width apart with your arms hanging straight down at your sides.

2. With your back straight, slowly squat down until your butt just touches the bench—the bench should be at a height high enough so that your butt touches it when your thighs are just short of being parallel to the floor.

3. Immediately push yourself back up into a standing position.

Note: If your bench is too low, just put a pillow, a folded-up towel, etc., on the bench so your butt touches the bench sooner as you squat. You're not placing your weight on the bench—touching it is just meant to remind you to stop squatting and reverse the motion.

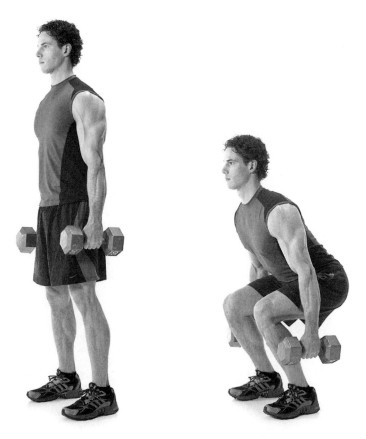

Squat

1. Stand straight holding a dumbbell in each hand and your feet spaced hip-width apart, knees unlocked.

2. Let your arms hang straight down at your sides, palms facing in.

3. Keeping your torso straight, slowly bend your knees and squat down until your thighs are parallel to the floor. (*Note:* Your knees should be directly above your toes—if they track forward past your toes, this can place unnecessary stress on your knees.)

4. Slowly stand back up—pressing through your heels, not your toes, as you go—until your legs are straight, knees unlocked.

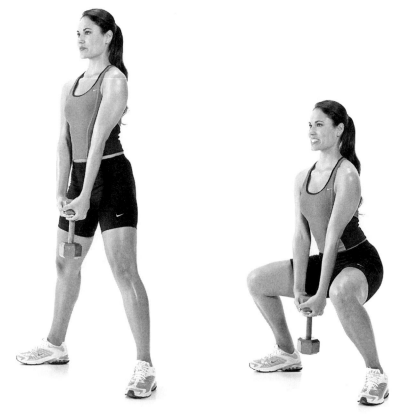

Sumo Squat

1. Stand with your feet slightly wider than shoulder-width apart, feet pointed out to the sides. Grab a heavy dumbbell by one end with both hands and let your arms hang down in front of you—the weight should be between your legs.

2. With your back straight, slowly squat down until your thighs are parallel to the floor.

3. Push yourself back up into a standing position, knees unlocked.

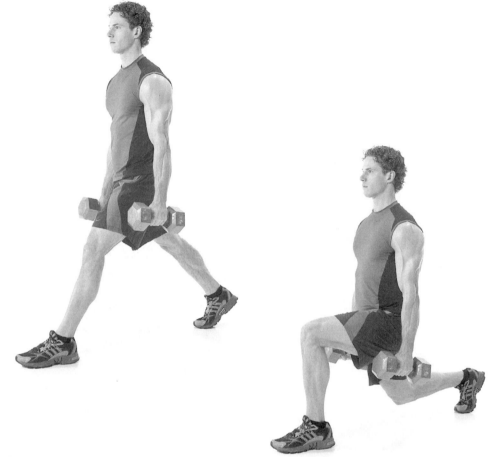

Split Squat

1. Stand holding a dumbbell in each hand, then step forward with your left foot and place it about 3 feet in front of your right foot. Your left foot will be flat on the floor, whereas your right foot will have only the ball of your foot touching the floor—your heel will be slightly elevated.

2. Holding this position, slowly squat down until your left thigh is parallel to the floor—your right knee should naturally lower down to just above the floor.

3. Press yourself back up and finish the required amount of reps. Then switch positions—placing your right foot forward—and repeat the exercise for the required amount of reps.

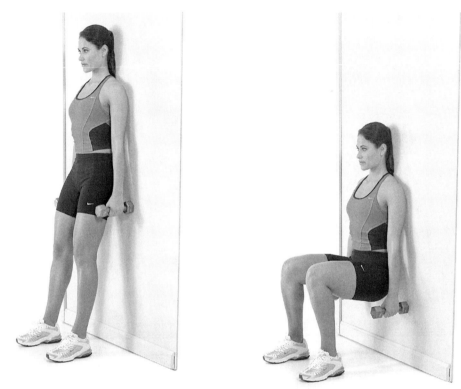

Wall Squat

1. Stand about 18 to 24 inches away from a sturdy wall, with your back facing the wall and a dumbbell in each hand.

2. Lean back into the wall so that your head, back, and butt are resting against it.

3. Bend your legs and slowly slide down the wall until your thighs are almost parallel to the floor.

4. Press yourself back up until your legs are straight—knees unlocked—and repeat the required amount of reps.

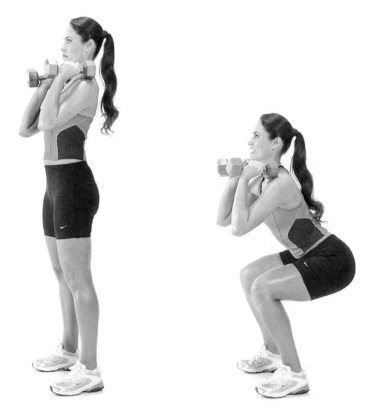

Front Squat

1. Stand straight holding a dumbbell in each hand and your feet spaced hip-width apart.

2. Raise both dumbbells up to your chest and place the ends of each dumbbell on the front of your shoulders—your palms will be facing in toward each other, elbows pointing down.

3. Follow Steps 3–4 of the Squat (see page 184).

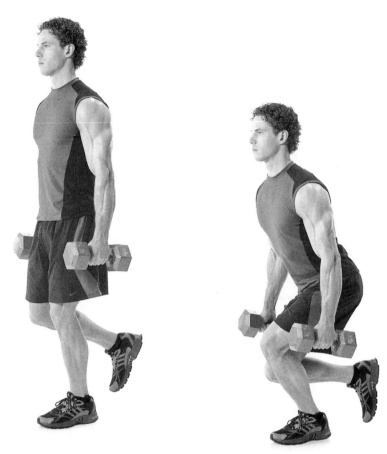

Single-Leg Squat

1. Stand straight, holding a dumbbell in each hand with your feet spaced hip-width apart. Bend your right knee and raise your right foot up behind you and hold it there.

2. Keeping your balance, slowly squat down until your left thigh is almost parallel to the floor.

3. Push yourself back up into a standing position, then repeat the exercise with your right leg by lowering your right foot back down to the floor and raising your left foot up behind you. Then squat down until your right thigh is almost parallel to the floor. Alternate from left to right for the entire set.

Multiply Your Moves! Beginner

There are *seven* versions of the squat. Here are a few different variations to try to keep things interesting.

Halfway Squat (creates 7 "new" moves!) Instead of squatting down until your thighs are parallel to the floor, lower yourself down only about half the distance, then stand back up—your butt will lower only about 5 to 7 inches. The shorter distance may not seem like much, but it offers most of the same benefits without being as stressful on the knees or requiring as much balance to perform.

Multiply Your Moves! Intermediate

Overhead Press (creates 6 "new" moves!) Instead of letting the weights hang down at your sides, raise the dumbbells over your head and keep them there as you squat. *Note:* You can use this with all of the squats, except the Single-Leg Squat—it's too difficult to stay balanced.

Multiply Your Moves! Intermediate "Plus"

Reverse Halfway Squat (creates 7 "new" moves!) Start the exercise by squatting down until your thighs are almost parallel to the floor. But instead of pushing yourself back up into a standing position, rise up only about half the distance. Continue to squat all the way down—so your thighs are parallel to the floor—then push yourself up half the distance for the entire set.

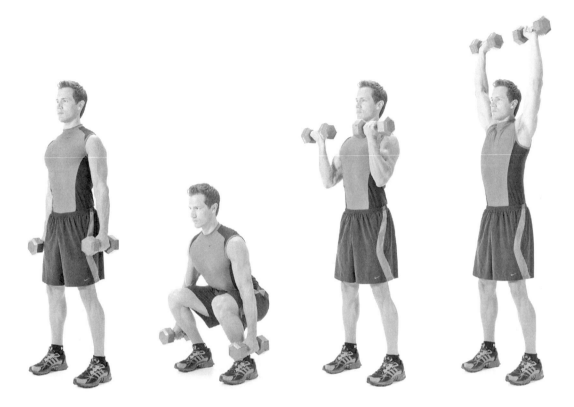

Curling Press Squat

(WORKS THE LEGS, GLUTEAL MUSCLES, LOWER BACK, BICEPS,
SHOULDERS, TRICEPS, CHEST, FOREARMS, ABDOMINALS, AND CALVES)

1. Stand straight with a dumbbell in each hand—palms facing in—with your feet shoulder-width apart.

2. Bend your knees, squat down until your thighs are almost parallel to the floor, and then stand back up.

3. Curl the weights up to your shoulders, twisting your wrists outward as you go—your palms should face your shoulders at the top.

4. Press the weights up over your head, twisting your wrists in 180 degrees so your palms face forward at the top.

5. Reverse the order of the exercise—lowering the weights, then curling them back down—until the weights are back down by your sides.

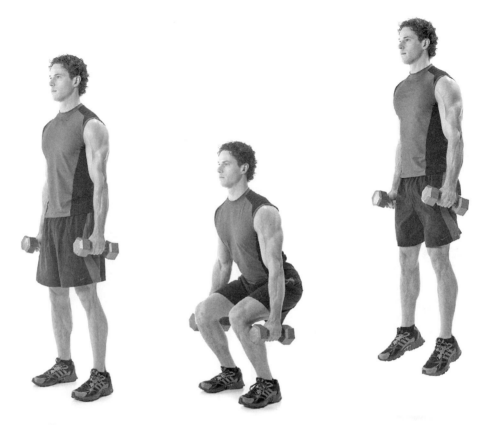

Squat Jump

(WORKS THE ENTIRE LOWER BODY)

1. Stand with a light dumbbell in each hand—feet slightly wider than shoulder-width apart—and your arms down at your sides.

2. With your head up, squat down until your thighs are parallel to the floor. Let your body lean forward slightly as you go.

3. Immediately jump straight up as high as you can, keeping your arms down along your sides.

4. Once your feet touch the floor, immediately squat back down. Continue to squat and jump for the entire set with no rest in between each jump.

EXERCISES FOR YOUR
SHOULDERS

≫BENT-OVER RAISE

This important exercise strengthens the always-neglected rear deltoids—the back of your shoulders—and the rotator cuff muscles; it also aids in drawing your shoulders back, which helps with posture and better breathing.

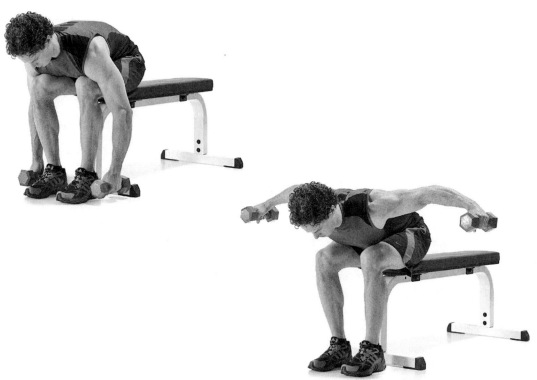

Bent-Over Raise

1. Sit on the edge of a bench—or an armless chair—with a light dumbbell in each hand.

2. Bending at the waist, lean forward until your chest touches your thighs—or as close as possible. Let your arms hang straight down below you, palms facing in toward each other.

3. Keeping your back fixed in this position and your arms straight, elbows unlocked, slowly raise the weights out to your sides until your arms are parallel to the floor.

4. Hold for a second, then slowly lower your arms back down until they're hanging directly below you once more.

Note: As you perform the exercise, try to keep your torso from moving. Lifting it up—even slightly—as you raise the weights uses momentum and your lower back instead of the muscles you're trying to work.

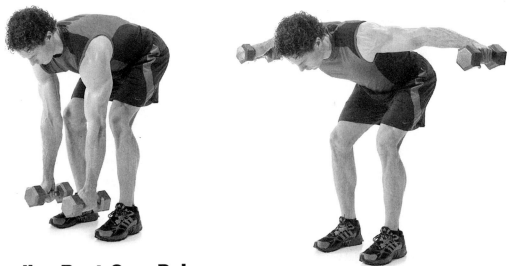

Standing Bent-Over Raise

1. Stand straight holding a light dumbbell in each hand.

2. Bending at the waist, lean forward until your back is flat and as parallel to the floor as possible—let your arms hang down directly below you, palms facing each other.

3. Follow Steps 3–4 of the Bent-Over Raise (see opposite page).

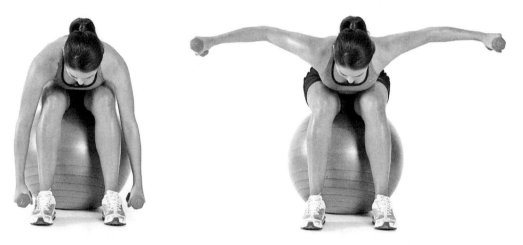

Swiss-Ball Bent-Over Raise

1. Sit on a Swiss ball with a light dumbbell in each hand. Keep your legs bent with your feet flat on the floor.

2. Follow Steps 2–4 of the Bent-Over Raise (see page 196).

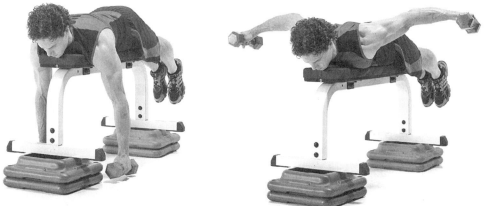

Lying Flat Bench Bent-Over Raise

1. Lie prone on an exercise bench with a light dumbbell in each hand.

2. Shimmy to the end of the bench so that your head hangs off and your neck is in line with your back—let your arms hang down below you, palms facing each other.

3. Follow Steps 3–4 of the Bent-Over Raise (see page 196).

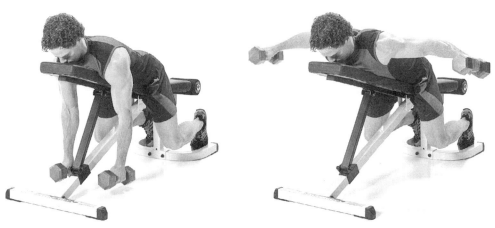

Lying Incline Bench Bent-Over Raise

1. Set an incline bench at a 30- to 45-degree angle, then grab a light dumbbell in each hand.

2. Sit backward on the bench with your chin, chest, and stomach flat against the pad—let your arms hang down below you, palms facing each other.

3. Follow Steps 3–4 of the Bent-Over Raise (see page 196).

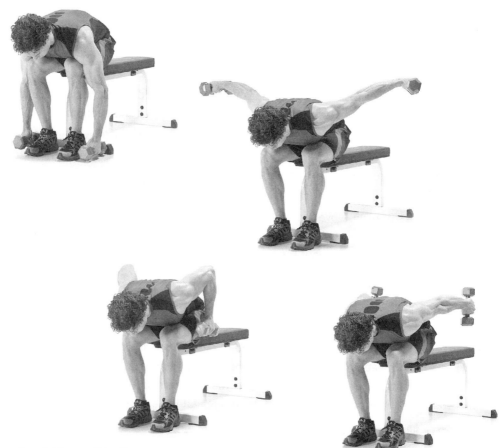

Seated Row/Raise

(WORKS YOUR BACK, TRICEPS, AND REAR SHOULDERS)

1. Sit on the edge of a bench—or an armless chair—with a light dumbbell in each hand. Bend at the waist and lean forward until your chest touches your thighs. Let your arms hang straight down below you, palms facing each other.

2. Raise the weights out to your sides until your arms are parallel to the floor.

3. Lower your arms back down, then row the weights up to your sides.

4. Keeping your upper arms parallel to your torso, straighten both arms behind you.

5. Bend your elbows and lower the weights back to the sides of your chest, then lower your arms back down until they're hanging straight down once again.

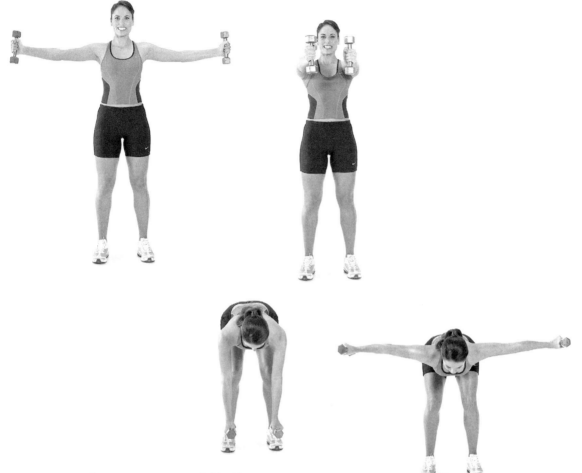

Three-Stage Lateral Raise

(WORKS ALL THREE SIDES OF YOUR SHOULDERS—FRONT, SIDE, AND REAR—
AND THE LOWER BACK)

1. Stand straight with a light dumbbell in each hand and raise your arms straight out to your sides, palms facing forward.

2. Keeping your arms straight, swing them in front of you until your hands are shoulder-width apart, palms facing each other.

3. Bend at the waist until your back is parallel to the floor; your arms should hang straight down, palms in.

4. Keeping your back parallel, extend your arms out to your sides.

5. Raise back up into a standing position.

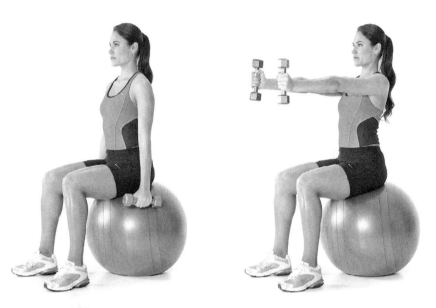

Swiss-Ball Front Raise

1. Sit on a Swiss ball with a light dumbbell in each hand. Keep your legs together; feet flat on the floor.

2. Your hands should be hanging down at your sides, with your palms facing back behind you.
Follow Steps 3–4 of the Front Raise (see page 204).

Note: If you find it difficult to position your hands with your palms facing backward—
a problem that people with narrower shoulders tend to experience—turn your palms in
toward the ball instead (as shown).

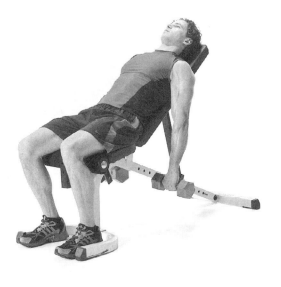

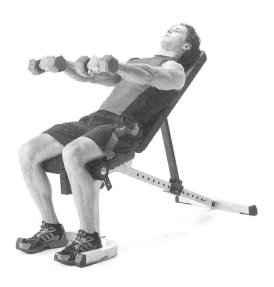

Lying Incline Bench Front Raise

1. Set an incline bench at a 45-degree angle, then grab a light dumbbell in each hand.

2. Sit on the bench and let your arms hang straight down, palms facing behind you—your arms should be angled slightly behind your torso.

3. Follow Steps 3–4 of the Front Raise (see page 204).

Multiply Your Moves! Intermediate "Plus"

Create your own hybrid exercise by doing a beginner variation and an intermediate move. You'll perform exercises that ask for your muscle's undivided attention.

One Arm at a Time + Neutral Grip (creates 6 "new" moves!) Before you start, twist your wrists in so that your palms face each other. Then, keep them in this position as you raise and lower the weights one arm at a time.

One Arm at a Time + Add a Twist (creates 12 "new" moves!) Try any of the 12 versions created by adding either type of twist, but up the intensity by doing the exercise one arm at a time.

One Up, One Down + Neutral Grip (creates 6 "new" moves!) Before you start, twist your wrists in so that your palms face each other. Then, keep them in this position as you raise one weight as you lower the other.

One Up, One Down + Add a Twist (creates 12 "new" moves!) Try any of the 12 versions created by adding either type of twist, but make it more of a challenge by raising the weight in one hand as you lower the weight in the other.

Multiply Your Moves! Advanced

Unbalanced Grip (creates 144 "new" moves!) Every Master Move in this section—including all 66 variations—have you holding the dumbbells in the center of the handle. Instead, try sliding your hands either all the way to the left or the right of the handle. Look at your hands and they will be in one of two positions:

» The thumb side of your hand(s) will be pressed against the inside plate of the dumbbell(s).

» The pinky side of your hand(s) will be pressed against the inside plate of the dumbbell(s).

The weights will feel off-center in your hands, no matter which way you choose to slide your hands. This places even more stress on your shoulder muscles for greater development.

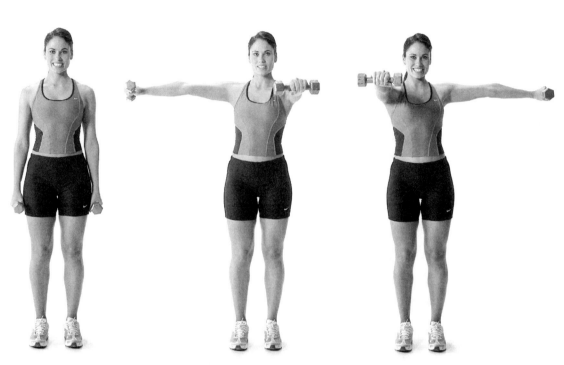

Unilateral Front/Side Raise

(WORKS THE FRONT AND SIDE DELTOIDS)

1. Stand with a light dumbbell in each hand, palms facing in.

2. Keeping your arms perfectly straight, slowly raise the weight in your left hand out and up in front of you until your left arm is parallel to the floor. Simultaneously raise your right arm out to your side until it's parallel to the floor.

3. Lower both arms down, then repeat the exercise, this time raising your right arm in front of you as you raise your left arm straight to the side.

4. Keep alternating between Steps 2 and 3 for the remainder of the set.

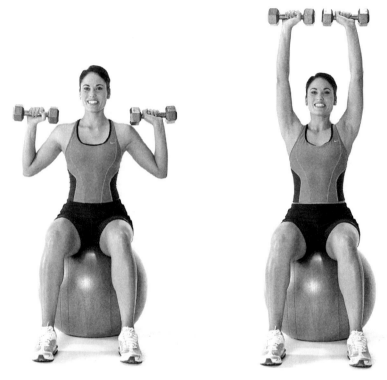

Swiss-Ball Shoulder Press

1. Sit on top of a Swiss ball with your feet flat on the floor and a dumbbell in each hand.

2. Follow Steps 2–4 of the Seated Shoulder Press (see page 212).

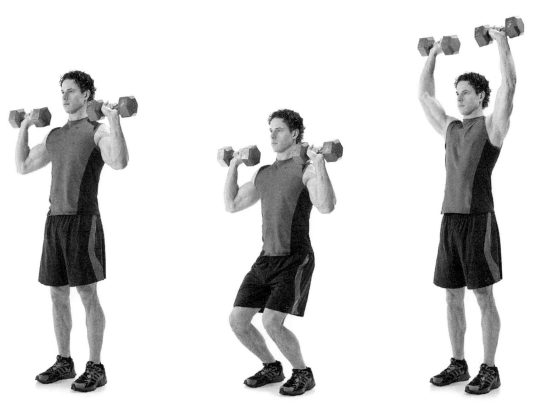

Push Press

1. Stand straight with your feet shoulder-width apart and a dumbbell in each hand.

2. Bring the weights up to the sides of your shoulders—elbows pointing down, palms facing forward.

3. Holding this position, immediately squat down a few inches, then push yourself back up into a standing position as you press the weights overhead.

4. Slowly lower the weights back down to your shoulders.

Multiply Your Moves! Beginner

Although there are only *four* basic versions of the Shoulder Press, there are 95 variations at your disposal. Here's how to get started!

All four versions of the Shoulder Press have you angle your palms facing forward. Instead, try these with any exercise in this section.

Neutral Grip (creates 4 "new" moves!) Before you start, twist your wrists in so that your palms face in toward each other. Then, keep them in this position as you press and lower the weights.

Underhand Grip (creates 4 "new" moves!) Before you start, twist your wrists so that your palms face in toward your shoulders. Then, keep them in this position as you press and lower the weights.

Add a Twist (creates 24 "new" moves!)

If you're starting the exercise in the traditional way—palms facing forward—twist the dumbbells out as you press them overhead, either:

>> 90 degrees—so your palms face each other at the top.

>> 180 degrees—so your knuckles face forward at the top.

If you're starting the exercise with a neutral grip—palms facing each other—twist the dumbbells as you press them overhead, either:

>> In—so your palms face forward at the top.

>> Out—so your knuckles face forward at the top.

If you're starting the exercise with an underhand grip—knuckles facing forward—twist the dumbbells in as you press them overhead, either:

>> 90 degrees—so your palms face each other at the top.

>> 180 degrees—so your palms face forward at the top.

No matter which version you try, reverse the motion as you lower the weights back down so your palms return to their original position when above you.

Multiply Your Moves! Intermediate

One Arm at a Time (creates 4 "new" moves!) Instead of pressing both weights simultaneously, try pressing up the weight in your left arm first, keeping the weight in your right hand down by your shoulder. Lower your left arm back down, then repeat the exercise, this time pressing the weight in your right arm up while keeping your left arm stationary. Alternate from left to right throughout the exercise.

One Up, One Down (creates 3 "new" moves!) Instead of pressing up both weights, press the one in your left hand first. As you lower the weight back down, simultaneously press the weight in your right hand up. Continue the exercise by pressing one weight as you lower the other for the entire set. *Note: This variation doesn't work with the Push Press.*

Multiply Your Moves! Intermediate "Plus"

If you've ever seen a unique shoulder press exercise, chances are it's one of the variations you can create mixing a beginner variation with an intermediate variation. Take your time trying these equilibrium-taxing, muscle-building moves.

One Arm at a Time + Neutral Grip (creates 4 "new" moves!) Before you start, twist your wrists in so that your palms face each other. Then, keep them in this position as you press and lower the weights one arm at a time.

One Arm at a Time + Underhand Grip (creates 4 "new" moves!) Before you start, twist your wrists in so that your knuckles face forward. Then, keep them in this position as you press and lower the weights one arm at a time.

One Arm at a Time + Add a Twist (creates 24 "new" moves!) Try any of the 24 versions created by adding any of the six types of twists, but up the intensity by doing the exercise one arm at a time.

One Up, One Down + Neutral Grip (creates 3 "new" moves!) Before you start, twist your wrists in so that your palms face each other. Then, keep them in this position as you press one weight as you lower the other. *Note: This variation—and the other two below—do not work with the Push Press.*

One Up, One Down + Underhand Grip (creates 3 "new" moves!) Before you start, twist your wrists in so that your knuckles face forward. Then, keep them in this position as you press one weight as you lower the other.

One Up, One Down + Add a Twist (creates 18 "new" moves!) Try any of the versions created by adding any of the six types of twists, but make it more of a challenge by pressing the weight in one hand as you lower the weight in the other. *Note: This variation is too difficult to do with the Push Press.*

Multiply Your Moves! Advanced

Unbalanced Grip (creates 198 "new" moves!) All four exercises in this section—including all 95 variations—have you holding the dumbbells in the center of the handle. Instead, try sliding your hands either all the way to the left or the right of the handle. Look at your hands and they will be in one of two positions:

» The thumb side of your hand(s) will be pressed against the inside plate of the dumbbell(s).

» The pinky side of your hand(s) will be pressed against the inside plate of the dumbbell(s).

The weights will feel off-center in your hands, no matter which way you choose to slide your hands. Your shoulders will rely on additional muscle fibers they typically don't use during regular-grip presses.

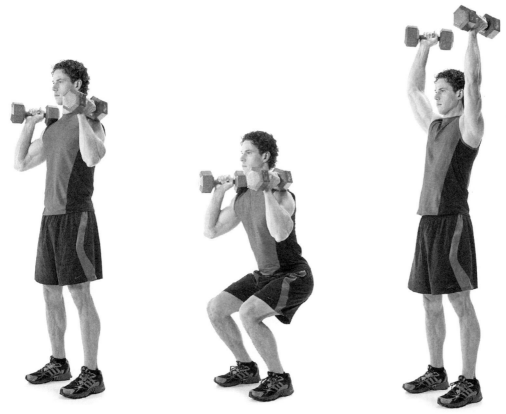

Shoulder Press Squat

(WORKS THE SHOULDERS AND LOWER BODY)

1. Stand straight with your feet shoulder-width apart, holding a dumbbell in each hand. Bring the weights up to the sides of your shoulders and rest the ends on your shoulders—your elbows should point down with your palms facing in.

2. Maintaining this posture, slowly bend your knees and squat down until your thighs are almost parallel to the floor.

3. Quickly stand up as you simultaneously press the weights up—you should end up in a standing position with the weights above your head.

4. Lower the weights back down to the fronts of your shoulders.

≫SIDE RAISE

This single-joint exercise isolates the medial deltoids—the muscle head that forms the sides of your shoulders.

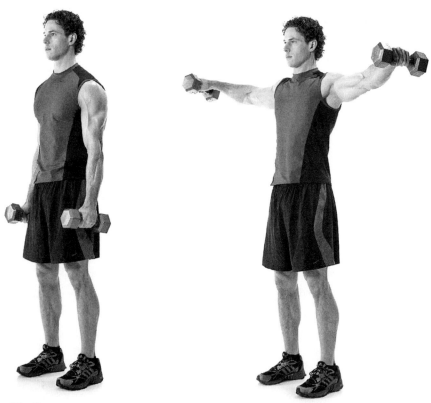

Basic Side Raise

1. Stand with a light dumbbell in each hand, your arms straight down at your sides.

2. Turn the weights so that your palms face in toward each other.

3. Keeping your arms straight, elbows unlocked, slowly raise the weights out and away from your body until your arms are parallel to the floor.

4. Hold for a second, then slowly lower your arms back down.

Note: Avoid bringing the dumbbells in front of your body so they clink together. This alters the angle, drawing in more muscles from the front portion of your shoulder (your anterior deltoids) and less of the muscles you're trying to work (the medial deltoids which make up the sides of your shoulders).

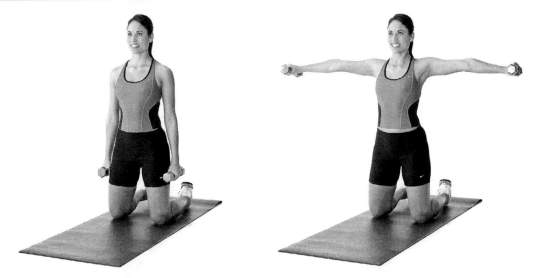

Kneeling Side Raise

1. Get into a kneeling position with a dumbbell in each hand, arms at your sides. Your back should be straight and in line with your thighs.

2. Follow Steps 2–4 of the Basic Side Raise (see opposite page).

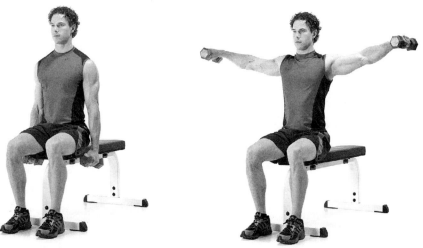

Seated Side Raise

1. Sit on the edge of a bench—or an armless chair—with a light dumbbell in each hand and your arms hanging straight down at your sides.

2. Follow Steps 2–4 of the Basic Side Raise (see opposite page).

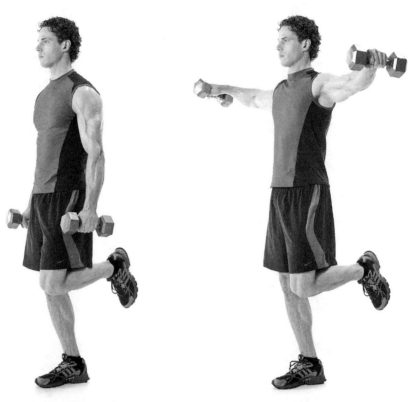

Single-Leg Lateral Raise

1. Stand as you would to do the Basic Side Raise—arms at your sides holding a dumbbell in each hand. Bend your left leg and raise your left foot up slightly behind you so you're balancing on your right foot only.

2. Follow Steps 2–4 of the Basic Side Raise (see page 220) for the entire set. Afterward, switch positions and balance on your left foot for the next set.

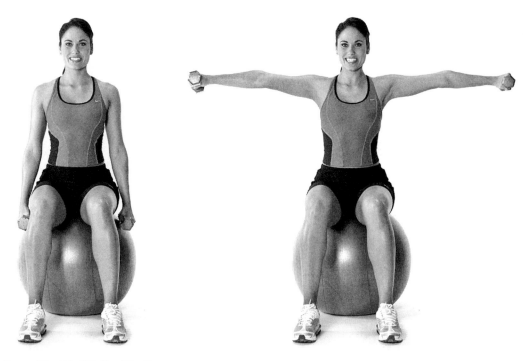

Swiss-Ball Side Raise

1. Sit on a Swiss ball with a light dumbbell in each hand and your arms hanging straight down at your sides. Spread your legs slightly and place your feet flat on the floor for stability.

2. Follow Steps 2–4 of the Basic Side Raise (see page 220).

Multiply Your Moves! Beginner

While there are 7 versions of the Side Raise in this section, you can perform at least 66 beginner and intermediate variations with these simple-to-do tweaks.

Every version of the Side Raise has you angle your palms in toward each other at the start of the exercise. Instead, try either of these two tweaks with any exercise in this section.

Overhand Grip (creates 7 "new" moves!) Before you start the exercise, twist your wrists in so that your knuckles face forward. Then keep them in this position as you perform the move; your palms should stay facing behind you throughout the entire exercise. *Note:* This tweak forces your rear deltoids to help raise the weights.

Underhand Grip (creates 7 "new" moves!) Before you start the exercise, twist your wrists outward so that your palms face forward. Then keep them in this position as you perform the move; your palms should stay facing forward throughout the entire exercise. *Note:* This tweak causes your front deltoids to help lift the weights.

Multiply Your Moves! Intermediate

One Arm at a Time (creates 5 "new" moves!) Instead of raising both arms at the same time, raise your left arm only, then lower it. Repeat the exercise, this time raising just your right arm out to the side. Alternate from left to right throughout the exercise. *Note:* This tweak won't work with the Intermediate "Plus" Master Moves, because they already have you working each arm separately.

One Up, One Down (creates 5 "new" moves!) Instead of raising both weights, try raising your left arm first. As you lower your arm back down, simultaneously raise your right arm. Continue the exercise by lowering one arm as you raise the other arm for the entire set. *Note:* This tweak also doesn't work with the Intermediate "Plus" Master Moves.

Add a Twist (creates 42 "new" moves!)

If you're starting the exercise in the traditional way—palms facing each other—twist the dumbbells either:

» In—so your palms face behind you at the top.

» Out—so your palms face forward at the top.

If you're starting the exercise with an overhand grip—knuckles facing forward—twist the dumbbells out either:

» 90 degrees—so your palms face down at the top.

» 180 degrees—so your palms face forward at the top.

If you're starting the exercise with an underhand grip—palms facing forward—twist the dumbbells in either:

» 90 degrees—so your palms face down at the top.

» 180 degrees—so your knuckles face forward at the top.

No matter which version you try, reverse the motion as you lower the weights back down so they return to their original position.

Multiply Your Moves! Intermediate "Plus"

Five of the Master Moves turn into 80 more when you combine a few variations in the right way. *Note:* These tweaks work only with the Beginner and Intermediate Master Moves—which have you use both arms.

One Arm at a Time + Overhand Grip (creates 5 "new" moves!) Before you start, twist your wrists in so that your knuckles face forward. Then keep them in this position as you raise and lower the weights one arm at a time.

One Arm at a Time + Underhand Grip (creates 5 "new" moves!) Before you start, twist your wrists out so that your palms face forward. Then keep them in this position as you raise and lower the weights one arm at a time.

One Arm at a Time + Add a Twist (creates 30 "new" moves!) Try any of the 30 two-arm versions created by adding any of the six types of twists, but up the intensity by doing the exercise one arm at a time.

One Up, One Down + Overhand Grip (creates 5 "new" moves!) Before you start, twist your wrists in so that your knuckles face forward. Then, keep them in this position as you raise one weight as you lower the other.

One Up, One Down + Underhand Grip (creates 5 "new" moves!) Before you start, twist your wrists out so that your palms face forward. Then, keep them in this position as you raise one weight as you lower the other.

One Up, One Down + Add a Twist (creates 30 "new" moves!) Try any of the 30 two-arm versions created by adding any of the six types of twists, but make it more of a challenge by raising the weight in one hand as you lower the weight in the other.

Multiply Your Moves! Advanced

These three tiny tweaks are subtle, but they can be used with every Master Move and all 146 variations to create 612 more shoulder-shaping exercises.

Butt Touch (creates 153 "new" moves!) Instead of lowering your arms straight down to your sides, try drawing your arms back 1 or 2 inches so the dumbbells end up touching the edges of your butt.

This small angle change makes your rear shoulders help out with each rep—these tiny muscles are usually neglected by many exercisers, but they're vital if you're hoping to build a pair of well-balanced shoulders.

Stop 6 Inches Away (creates 153 "new" moves!) Instead of lowering your arms all the way down to your sides after each rep—so they hang straight down—try stopping the weights about 6 inches away from your legs. (You'll still raise them up so they're parallel to the floor as usual.)

Not dropping your arms all the way down places constant stress on your shoulders, forcing them to recruit even more muscle fibers than usual. *Note:* You may need to reduce the weight you typically use by 30 to 50 percent.

Unbalanced Grip (creates 306 "new" moves!) All seven exercises in this section—including all 146 variations up until now—have you holding the dumbbells in the center of the handle. Instead, try sliding your hands either all the way to the left or the right of the handle. Look at your hands and they will be in one of two positions:

» The thumb side of your hand(s) will be pressed against the inside plate of the dumbbell(s).

» The pinky side of your hand(s) will be pressed against the inside plate of the dumbbell(s).

The weights will feel off-center in your hands, no matter which way you choose to slide your hands. This makes your medial deltoids recruit more muscle fibers to stabilize the weights as you raise and lower them.

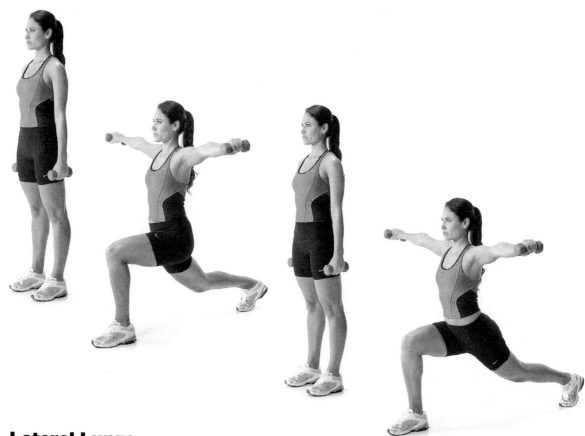

Lateral Lunge

(WORKS YOUR SHOULDERS, LEGS, AND CORE MUSCLES)

1. Stand as you would to do a side raise—arms at your sides holding a dumbbell in each hand.

2. Take a big step forward with your left foot and plant it flat on the floor. Lower your body until your left leg is bent at a 90-degree angle—knee over your toes.

3. As you lunge forward, simultaneously extend your arms out to your sides until your arms are parallel to the floor.

4. Push yourself back into a standing position as you simultaneously lower your arms back down to your sides.

5. Repeat the exercise, this time by stepping forward with your right foot.

»ADDITIONAL SHOULDER EXERCISES

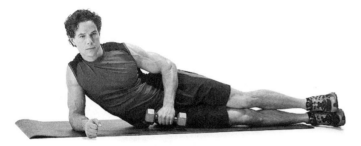

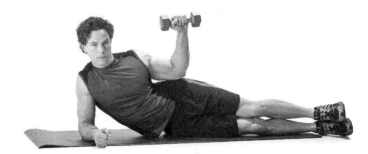

Lying Shoulder Rotation
(WORKS THE ROTATOR CUFF MUSCLES)

1. Lie on your right side with your legs and feet together, knees slightly bent for support. Bend your right arm at a 90-degree angle and rest your elbow and forearm on the floor, fist pointing forward. Grab a very light dumbbell in your left hand and position your left arm so that your upper arm is flat against your side, arm bent at 90 degrees with the dumbbell hanging in front of your stomach.

2. Without moving your upper arm, rotate your arm and raise the weight up until it's directly above your left elbow—your arm should still be bent at 90 degrees.

3. Reverse the motion by rotating the weight back down, finish the set, then switch positions to work your right arm.

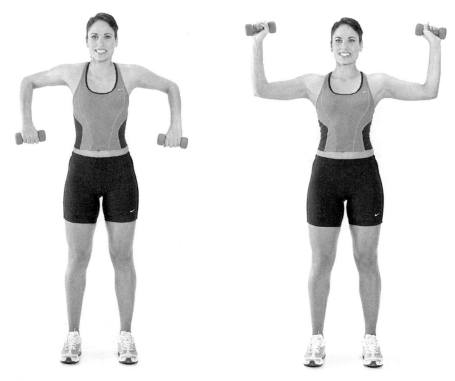

Standing Shoulder Rotation

(WORKS THE ROTATOR CUFF MUSCLES)

1. Stand straight with a very light dumbbell in each hand. Raise your elbows out to the sides until your upper arms are parallel to the floor with the weights pointing down—your arms should be bent at 90-degree angles.

2. Without moving your upper arms, rotate your arms and raise the weights forward until they are directly above your elbows—your arms should still be bent at 90 degrees.

3. Reverse the motion by rotating the weights back down.

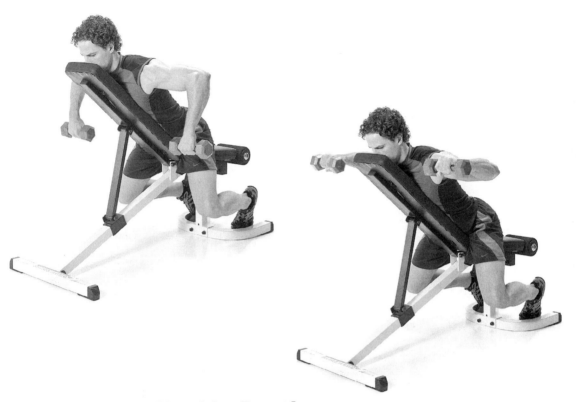

Incline Bench Shoulder Rotation

(WORKS THE ROTATOR CUFF MUSCLES)

1. Set an incline bench at a 45-degree angle, grab a very light dumbbell in each hand, and sit backward on the bench. Your chest and stomach should rest flat against the backrest.

2. Raise your elbows out to the sides until your upper arms are parallel to the floor with the weights pointing down—your arms should be bent at 90-degree angles.

3. Without moving your upper arms, rotate your arms and raise the weights forward until your forearms are parallel to the floor—your arms should still be bent at 90 degrees.

4. Reverse the motion by rotating the weights back down.

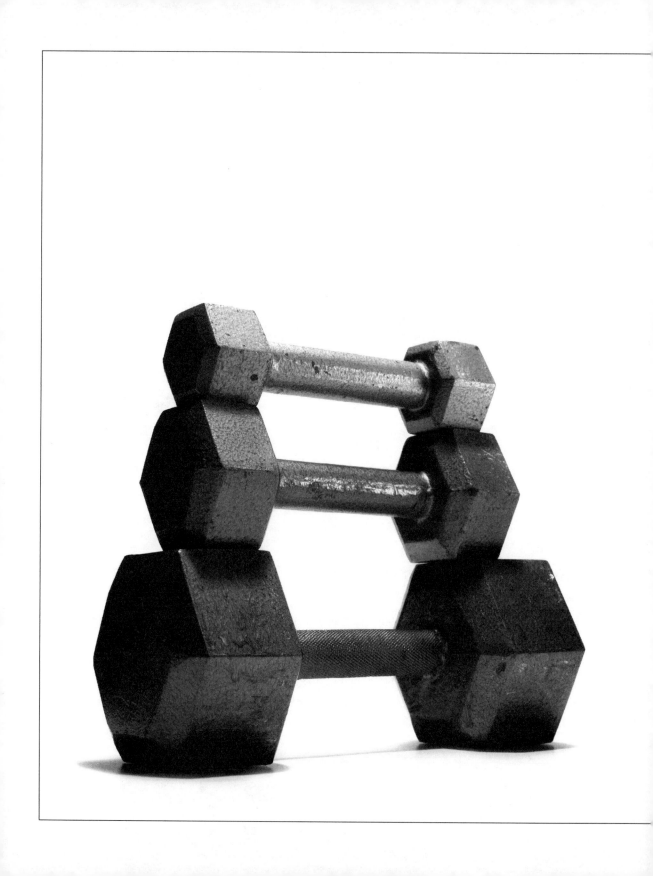

PART THREE

A MILLION MOVES FOR YOUR MUSCLES

TRY THIS TRICK WITH EVERY EXERCISE IN THIS BOOK

Beginner

Continuous Contraction
(Creates 4,988 New Exercises!)

This tweak is perfect for beginners because it teaches you to feel the muscles you're trying to train "before" and "during" the exercise. Don't worry that you can't lift as much weight. The point of any exercise is to exhaust your muscles to force them to change, and this tweak lets you accomplish just that using less weight.

Before you start any exercise, flex the muscles you're about to work and keep flexing them as you perform the exercise. *Note:* Don't worry if some exercises won't allow you to keep your muscles flexed the entire time—just do your best.

Intermediate

Do Three Mini-Reps
(Creates 4,988 New Exercises!)

Using this trick with every exercise forces you to keep the muscles you're training contracted longer, so you end up recruiting even more muscle fibers than usual for greater improvements.

Each time you raise the weight, avoid the urge to lower it back down immediately. Instead, perform three "mini-reps"—lowering the weight just 1 to 2 inches—in between each normal repetition.

Intermediate "Plus"

Wait 3 Seconds
(Creates 4,988 New Exercises!)

This tweak can take the tamest exercise and turn it into a brutal move that pushes your muscles to new limits. This is especially true of exercises where many people tend to use momentum to help cheat the weight up. This tactic also makes you start every single repetition fresh, so there's less chance of your raising the weight with other muscles besides the ones you want to work. However, you may want to use less weight than usual—20 to 30 percent—when using it.

Instead of immediately raising the dumbbells each time you lower them back down, wait and hold them at the bottom for exactly 3 seconds.

■ If it's an exercise where your arms end up down at your sides, like biceps curls and front or side raises, for example, keep the weights about an inch away from your legs so there's tension on your muscles while you wait.

■ If it's an exercise where your arms end up directly beneath you—bent-over raises, bent-over rows, etc.—then stop about an inch away from the bottom of the move to keep tension on the muscles.

■ If it's a leg exercise—squat, lunge, etc.— stop at the bottom of the move instead (where you're either squatting or lunging). This maneuver can be extremely difficult to perform with leg exercises, but you'll achieve terrific results if you use it. Beginners may find this tweak too challenging because of the balance it requires, so ease into it by pausing 1 second to start, then work your way up to 3 seconds over time.

TRY THIS TRICK WITH EVERY STANDING-STRAIGHT EXERCISE

Beginner–Intermediate

Raise Your Foot

(Creates 626 New Exercises!)

While this trick is either impossible or too risky to do with any of the exercises that work your legs, it is effective for most upper-body exercises like presses, curls, raises, rows, and so on. It allows you to improve your balance while you strengthen your leg muscles at the same time.

Instead of keeping both feet flat on the floor, try suspending one foot an inch above the floor so your weight is on the supporting foot throughout the exercise. After each set—or repetition, if you really want to try something unique—lower your foot back down and raise the opposite foot. Keep alternating back and forth between feet so you train them equally.

Intermediate "Plus"

Raise Your Heels

(Creates 626 New Exercises!)

Again, while this trick doesn't apply to any of the leg exercises in this book, it's very effective for exercises that work your upper body (presses, curls, raises, rows, extensions, and so on). You'll improve your overall balance while strengthening your calves.

Instead of keeping both feet flat on the floor, try raising both heels just off the floor so that your weight is on the balls of your feet as you perform the exercise. You can use this trick for the entire set, every other rep, or every other set.

TRY THIS TRICK WITH EVERY INCLINE-DECLINE BENCH EXERCISE

Beginner–Intermediate "Plus"

Raise/Lower After Every Set

(Creates 774 New Exercises!)

Whenever an exercise requires you to use an incline or decline bench, don't keep the backrest at the same angle for the entire exercise. Raising or lowering it with every set can train your muscles from several angles instead of just one.

Instead of setting the incline bench at the standard 45-degree angle, set it lower than that—a few inches from being completely flat. Do one set of whichever exercise you're performing, then raise the backrest one notch. Keep raising the backrest—one notch higher than the last—before you perform each set. *Note:* If you run out of notches toward the end, or end up with the backrest perpendicular to the floor, reverse the direction and start lowering the backrest one notch before performing each set.

The same rule applies to any decline-bench exercise. Start with the backrest one notch below its flat position. Do one set of whichever exercise you're performing, then lower the backrest one notch. Keep lowering the backrest—one notch lower than the last—before you perform each set. *Note:* If you run out of notches toward the end, reverse the direction and start raising it one notch instead.

Seven

CREATE YOUR OWN SPECIALTY DUMBBELL EXERCISE!

YOU'VE SEEN THEM. . . those interesting dumbbell exercises that magazines love to wow readers with. The ones that sometimes require a map to get you from point A to point B. The ones that feel more like learning how to dance or mastering a martial art than exercise, simply because of how many steps you're asked to perform. These are the ones that supposedly work several muscle groups at once, letting you work your entire body—or at least most of it—in less time, instead of wasting time isolating each muscle group separately.

I call them "multistep" moves—or specialty exercises.

You won't find that many "multistep" moves in this book—besides what I've shown you in the "Combine and Conquer" sections—but there's a reason for that. When broken down, many of these "all-in-one exercises" are really just a series of basic exercises—exercises you'll find in this book, actually—all strung together to create something that looks more unique than it really is.

Mind you, that doesn't mean these multistep exercises aren't effective in their own way. In fact, combining dumbbell exercises into one long exercise can be a terrific way to work more muscles simultaneously for a

faster full-body workout. They can also turn several otherwise anaerobic muscle-building exercises into one continuous aerobic routine, which is perfect if your main goal is improving your cardiovascular health, teaching your muscles to work together, and/or burning off excess body fat.

These multistep moves may seem difficult to perform, but they're not as hard to create as you may think. So instead of describing hundreds and hundreds of these multimove exercises, I'd rather give you the power to make them yourself. With this chapter, you can create any series of combination exercises you wish—whenever you need them—using many of the Master Moves you already know.

HOW IT WORKS

In this chapter, you'll see a series of boxes (labeled A through Q). Each box corresponds to the different positions your body gets placed in during exercise, with each box filled with all the exercise moves that you can do from that position. You'll start your exercise from a standing position—arms down at your sides—then pick a step from Box "A." Once you've chosen a step, it'll tell you which box to pick from next. It may be the same box, or it could be a different box—depending on what position your body ends up in after following the step you've chosen.

Numerically, there are thousands of exercise combinations you can make if you just string two to four steps together. But if you decide to combine five, six, seven, or even eight steps together, you can literally create *millions* and *millions* of different possible "multistep" exercises—just like the "Combine and Conquer" moves shown in this book.

CREATING YOUR MUSCLE MASTERPIECE!

Which steps should I pick, you may ask?

Each step in every box is labeled to let you know which muscle—or muscles—it works when you use it. You can choose to string together enough steps to create a full-body workout, or pick steps that focus on two or three muscle groups you think need more attention. You may also want to try picking them purely at random if you feel like doing something different every time you exercise. It's entirely up to you.

To design your own personal "multistep" dumbbell exercise:

■ Write down the starting position on a piece of paper (or photocopy the fill-in-the-blank list provided on page 242). Here is the starting position: *Stand straight with your feet shoulder-width apart and a light dumbbell in each hand.*

■ Next, select *one* step from the 18 options in Box "A," then write it down. Whichever step you choose, it will tell you at the end of the description which box to go to next to pick another step that works with the one you've just chosen.

■ Go to whichever box you've been told to go to next, pick another step, then write that down.

■ Keep adding steps in this way—from 3 to 8 steps total—until you feel you have enough in your exercise. Try to pick a final step that returns you to the starting position—standing straight with your arms at your sides.

Once you've created your exercise, name your move (why not? everyone else does!), then perform all the steps in the order given. Once you've run through all of the steps, repeat the cycle for as many repetitions as you can. Perform your "new" exercise for a total of two or three sets. *Note:* If the dumbbells you're using feel too light after you try the completed exercise, try increasing them by 1 to 2.5 pounds per dumbbell.

Make Your Personal "Multistep" Exercise Here

You already know Step #1. Now, just pick a step from Box "A" and see where it takes you next. Keep picking steps—as many as you like—then finish by choosing a final step that brings you back to choosing a step from Box "A" (this will bring you back into a standing position).

1. Stand straight with your feet shoulder-width apart and a light dumbbell in each hand.

2. _____

3. _____

4. _____

5. _____

6. _____

7. _____

8. _____

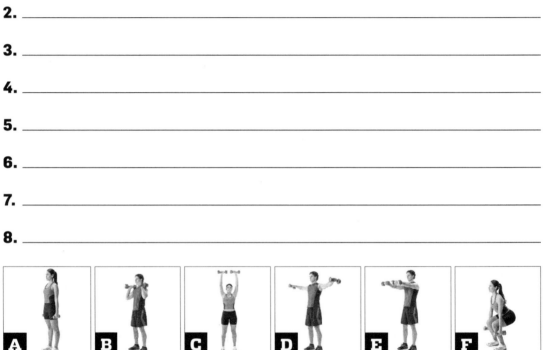

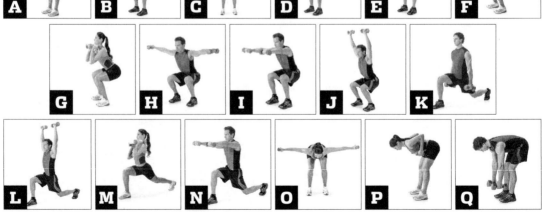

BOX "A"

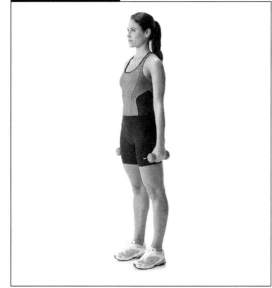

STANDING WITH ARMS DOWN AT YOUR SIDES

»(Abs/Obliques): Bend slightly to the left, then to the right **[GO TO BOX "A"]**

»(Back): Bend forward at the waist, letting your arms hang below you, then pull the weights up to the sides of your chest **[GO TO BOX "P"]**

»(Back + legs): Bend forward at the waist until your torso is parallel to the floor, letting the weights hang straight below you, then rise back into a standing position **[GO TO BOX "A"]**

»(Back + legs): Bend forward at the waist until your torso is parallel to the floor, letting the weights hang straight below you, then stay there **[GO TO BOX "Q"]**

»(Back + shoulders): Lift your shoulders up as high as you can—keeping your arms straight as you go—then lower them back down **[GO TO BOX "A"]**

»(Back): Pull the weights up close to your body until they are under your chin, then lower them back down **[GO TO BOX "A"]**

»(Biceps): Curl the weights up—palms facing up **[GO TO BOX "B"]**

»(Biceps): Curl the weights up—palms facing in **[GO TO BOX "B"]**

»(Biceps): Curl the weights up—palms facing down **[GO TO BOX "B"]**

»(Calves): Rise up on your toes, hold, then lower back down **[GO TO BOX "A"]**

»(Legs): Squat down until your thighs are parallel to the floor, then stay in that position **[GO TO BOX "F"]**

»(Legs): Squat down until your thighs are parallel to the floor, then stand back up **[GO TO BOX "A"]**

»(Legs): Lunge forward with your left foot, stand back up, repeat with your right foot, stand back up **[GO TO BOX "A"]**

»(Legs): Lunge backward with your left foot, stand back up, repeat with your right foot, stand back up **[GO TO BOX "A"]**

»(Legs): Lunge forward with your left foot, stand back up, repeat with your right foot, then stay in a lunge position **[GO TO BOX "K"]**

»(Legs): Lunge backward with your left foot, stand back up, repeat with your right foot, then stay in a lunge position **[GO TO BOX "K"]**

»(Shoulders): Raise your arms out to your sides **[GO TO BOX "D"]**

»(Shoulders): Raise your arms in front of you **[GO TO BOX "E"]**

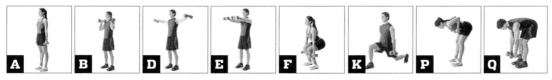

A   B   D   E   F   K   P   Q

BOX "D"

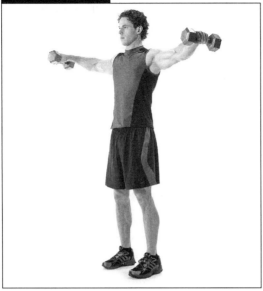

STANDING WITH ARMS EXTENDED OUT TO THE SIDES

»(Abs): Twist to the left and right **[GO TO BOX "D"]**

»(Biceps): Turn your palms up and curl the weights to your shoulders **[GO TO BOX "B"]**

»(Calves): Rise up on your toes, hold, then lower back down **[GO TO BOX "D"]**

»(Legs): Squat down until your thighs are parallel to the floor, then stay in that position **[GO TO BOX "H"]**

»(Legs): Squat down until your thighs are parallel to the floor, then stand back up **[GO TO BOX "D"]**

»(Legs): Lunge forward with your left foot, stand back up, repeat with your right foot, stand back up **[GO TO BOX "D"]**

»(Legs): Lunge backward with your left foot, stand back up, repeat with your right foot, stand back up **[GO TO BOX "D"]**

»(Legs): Lunge forward with your left foot, stand back up, repeat with your right foot, then stay in a lunge position **[GO TO BOX "M"]**

»(Legs): Lunge backward with your left foot, stand back up, repeat with your right foot, then stay in a lunge position **[GO TO BOX "M"]**

»(Shoulders): Lower the weights back down to your sides **[GO TO BOX "A"]**

»(Shoulders): Sweep your arms forward until your arms are in front of you **[GO TO BOX "E"]**

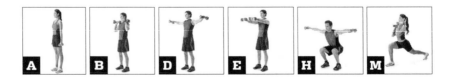

BOX "E"

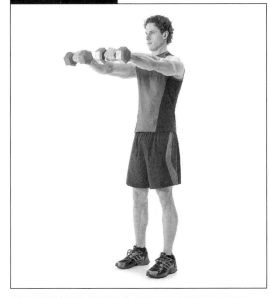

STANDING WITH ARMS EXTENDED IN FRONT OF YOU

»(Biceps + Shoulders): Without moving your upper arms, curl the weights toward your shoulders **[GO TO BOX "B"]**

»(Calves): Rise up on your toes, hold, then lower back down **[GO TO BOX "E"]**

»(Legs): Squat down until your thighs are parallel to the floor, then stay in that position **[GO TO BOX "I"]**

»(Legs): Squat down until your thighs are parallel to the floor, then stand back up **[GO TO BOX "E"]**

»(Legs): Lunge forward with your left foot, stand back up, repeat with your right foot, stand back up **[GO TO BOX "E"]**

»(Legs): Lunge backward with your left foot, stand back up, repeat with your right foot, stand back up **[GO TO BOX "E"]**

»(Legs): Lunge forward with your left foot, stand back up, repeat with your right foot, then stay in a lunge position **[GO TO BOX "N"]**

»(Legs): Lunge backward with your left foot, stand back up, repeat with your right foot, then stay in a lunge position **[GO TO BOX "N"]**

»(Shoulders): Lower the weights back down to your sides **[GO TO BOX "A"]**

»(Shoulders): Sweep your arms out to the sides **[GO TO BOX "D"]**

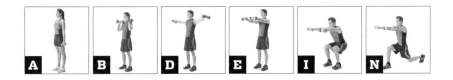

BOX "F"

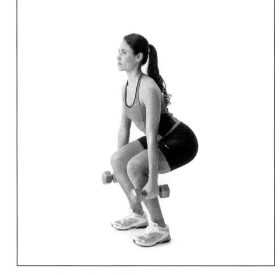

SQUATTING WITH ARMS DOWN AT YOUR SIDES

»(Back + shoulders): Lift your shoulders up as high as you can—keeping your arms straight as you go—then lower them back down **[GO TO BOX "F"]**

»(Biceps): Curl the weights up—palms facing up—then curl them back down **[GO TO BOX "F"]**

»(Biceps): Curl the weights up—palms facing in—then curl them back down **[GO TO BOX "F"]**

»(Biceps): Curl the weights up—palms facing down—then curl them back down **[GO TO BOX "F"]**

»(Biceps): Curl the weights up—palms facing up **[GO TO BOX "G"]**

»(Biceps): Curl the weights up—palms facing in **[GO TO BOX "G"]**

»(Biceps): Curl the weights up—palms facing down **[GO TO BOX "G"]**

»(Legs): Push back up into a standing position **[GO TO BOX "A"]**

»(Shoulders): Raise your arms out to your sides, then lower them **[GO TO BOX "F"]**

»(Shoulders): Raise your arms in front of you, then lower them **[GO TO BOX "F"]**

»(Triceps): Lean forward, extend your arms back behind you, then return to the starting position **[GO TO BOX "F"]**

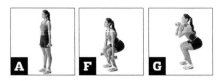

BOX "G"

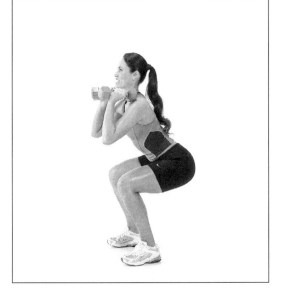

SQUATTING WITH WEIGHTS UP BY SHOULDERS

»(Biceps): Curl the weights back down to your sides **[GO TO BOX "F"]**

»(Legs): Push back up into a standing position **[GO TO BOX "B"]**

»(Shoulders): Push the weights overhead, then lower them back down **[GO TO BOX "G"]**

»(Shoulders): Push the weights overhead **[GO TO BOX "J"]**

BOX "H"

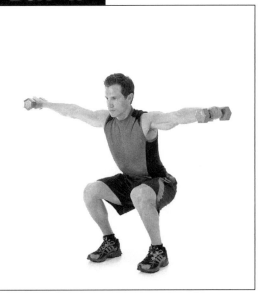

SQUATTING WITH ARMS EXTENDED OUT TO THE SIDES

»(Biceps + Shoulders): Without moving your upper arms, curl the weights toward your shoulders **[GO TO BOX "G"]**

»(Legs): Push back up into a standing position **[GO TO BOX "D"]**

»(Shoulders): Lower the weights back down to your sides **[GO TO BOX "F"]**

»(Shoulders): Sweep your arms forward until your arms are in front of you **[GO TO BOX "I"]**

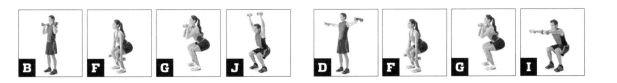

BOX "I"

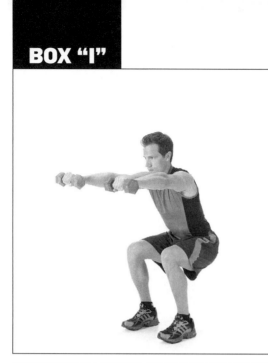

SQUATTING WITH ARMS EXTENDED IN FRONT OF YOU

»(Biceps + Shoulders): Without moving your upper arms, curl the weights toward your shoulders [GO TO BOX "G"]

»(Legs): Push back up into a standing position [GO TO BOX "E"]

»(Shoulders): Lower the weights back down to your sides [GO TO BOX "F"]

»(Shoulders): Sweep your arms out to the sides [GO TO BOX "H"]

BOX "J"

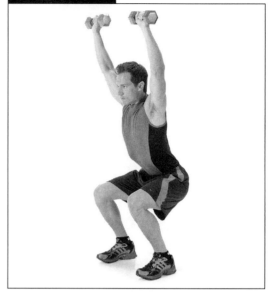

SQUATTING WITH WEIGHTS PRESSED OVERHEAD

»(Back + shoulders): Lift your shoulders up as high as you can—keeping your arms straight as you go—then lower them back down [GO TO BOX "J"]

»(Chest): Sweep your arms forward—palms facing each other—until your arms are back down at your sides [GO TO BOX "F"]

»(Legs): Push back up into a standing position [GO TO BOX "C"]

»(Shoulders): Lower the weights back down to your sides [GO TO BOX "F"]

»(Triceps): Turn your palms in towards each other, slowly bend your elbows and lower the weights behind your head, then press them back up [GO TO BOX "J"]

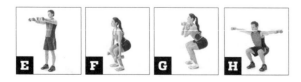

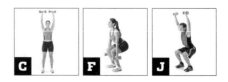

BOX "K"

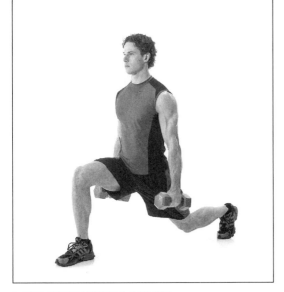

LUNGING WITH ARMS DOWN AT YOUR SIDES

>>**(Back + shoulders):** Lift your shoulders up as high as you can—keeping your arms straight as you go—then lower them back down **[GO TO BOX "K"]**

>>**(Biceps):** Curl the weights up—palms facing up—then curl them back down **[GO TO BOX "K"]**

>>**(Biceps):** Curl the weights up—palms facing in—then curl them back down **[GO TO BOX "K"]**

>>**(Biceps):** Curl the weights up—palms facing down—then curl them back down **[GO TO BOX "K"]**

>>**(Legs):** Push yourself back up into a standing position **[GO TO BOX "A"]**

>>**(Shoulders):** Raise your arms out to your sides, then lower them **[GO TO BOX "K"]**

>>**(Shoulders):** Raise your arms in front of you, then lower them **[GO TO BOX "K"]**

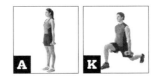

BOX "P"

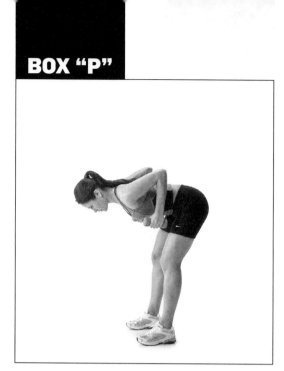

BENT OVER WITH WEIGHTS BY SIDES OF CHEST

»(Back): Raise your torso back up into a standing position, then lower your arms to your sides [GO TO BOX "A"]

»(Back): Lower the weights back down [GO TO BOX "Q"]

»(Triceps): Extend your arms straight back behind you, then return them to the starting position [GO TO BOX "P"]

BOX "Q"

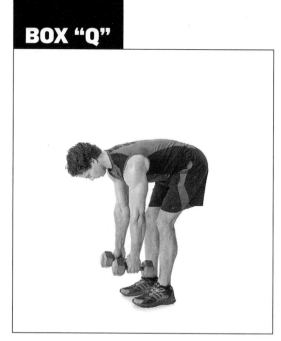

BENT OVER WITH ARMS HANGING STRAIGHT DOWN

»(Back): Raise your torso back up into a standing position [GO TO BOX "A"]

»(Back): Pull the weights up to the sides of your chest [GO TO BOX "P"]

»(Shoulders): Raise your arms out to the sides [GO TO BOX "O"]

»(Triceps): Extend your arms straight back behind you, then return them to the starting position [GO TO BOX "Q"]

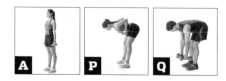

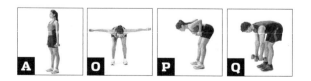

Eight

DESIGNING THE BEST PLAN FOR YOUR BODY!

YOU WOULD THINK THAT with so many options now at your disposal, attempting to instruct you on which exercises to use would be impossible.

Not so.

As I told you at the start of this book, it's the Master Moves that are some of the most effective exercises for building quality lean muscle and helping you reach your goals faster than you might expect. That's precisely why the routines in this section rely on nearly all of them to get that job done.

When using any and all of these routines, stick with the exercises recommended. After a few weeks, if you're looking to add a little variety or intensity to your workout, you can tweak an exercise—if possible—with the "Multiply Your Moves" options. Just remember to use only exercises, routines, and variations that match your current fitness level. Pushing yourself too soon—before your muscles are ready for change—won't help you see results any faster, but it will increase your risk of an injury.

REPS AND SETS

If you're following the routines in this section, you'll be told to perform each exercise for a certain amount of repetitions—or "reps." This means you should select a dumbbell that's heavy enough to exhaust the muscles you're trying to target within whatever required amount of reps you're instructed to perform. For example, if you're asked to do 12 to 15 reps, then you should choose a weight heavy enough so that your muscles can do that exercise only 12 to 15 times. If you can't do 12, then the weight is too heavy; if you can do more than 16, then the weight is too light.

The first few times you try a new exercise, you may spend a few sets figuring out the right amount of weight for you. In fact, you may waste a workout selecting the right weights the first few times you try a routine. That's entirely fine, so long as you write down how much weight was too light—or heavy—so you don't have to go through the same process the next time. Trust me, within one or two workouts, you'll discover the right amount of weight your muscles need to get a good workout from an exercise as described.

You'll also be told to perform each exercise for a certain amount of sets. This is the amount of times you'll repeat the exercise—doing whatever repetitions are required—before moving on to the next exercise in the order given.

BEGINNER WORKOUT #1

Hitting every muscle in your body in one shot doesn't take as much time as you might think. Arranging a plan that builds your upper and lower body in a single workout just requires using certain multifunctional exercises in the right order. The full-body routines you'll find in this section do just that—working larger muscles first and smaller secondary muscles last. That way, you'll always have enough energy to exhaust each muscle group thoroughly for maximum results.

Exercise	Muscles Worked	Page	Reps	Sets
Crunch	Upper abs	31	10–15	2
Reverse Crunch	Lower abs	32	10–15	2
Squat	Legs	183	10–12	2
Chest Press	Chest	148	10–12	3
Lunge	Legs	169	10–12	2
One-Arm Row	Back	106	10–12	2
Standing Shoulder Press	Shoulders	213	10–12	3
Pullover	Back	124	10–12	2
Biceps Curl	Biceps	45	10–12	2
Lying Extension	Triceps	75	10–12	2
Seated Calf Raise	Calves	162	10–12	2

» Rest 45–60 seconds between each set

» Perform this routine 2–3 times weekly

BEGINNER WORKOUT #2

Exercise	Muscles Worked	Page	Reps	Sets
Crunch	Upper abs	31	10–15	2
Reverse Crunch	Lower abs	32	10–15	2
Deadlift	Back, legs	116	10–12	3
Chest Press	Chest	148	10–12	3
Lunge	Legs	169	10–12	2
One-Arm Row	Back	106	10–12	2
Standing Shoulder Press	Shoulders	212	10–12	2
Biceps Curl	Biceps	45	10–12	1
Reverse Curl	Biceps	47	10–12	1
Lying Extension	Triceps	75	10–12	1
Two-Arm Extension	Triceps	94	10–12	1
Seated Calf Raise	Calves	162	10–12	2

» *Rest 45–60 seconds between each set*

» *Perform this routine 2–3 times weekly*

INTERMEDIATE WORKOUT #1

Having some experience under your belt gives you the option of exercising more than two or three times a week. However, breaking up your workouts so that you're working only certain muscles on certain days also lets you spend more time—and exercises—on each muscle group. All that extra attention can pay off with faster and more noticeable results.

ROUTINE A (ABS, LEGS, AND BACK)

Exercise	Muscles Worked	Page	Reps	Sets
Double Crunch	Abs	33	10–15	3
Cycle Crunch	Abs	34	10–15	3
Squat	Legs	183	10–15	4
Two-Arm Row	Back	104	10–15	3
Reverse Lunge	Legs	173	10–15	3
Stiff-Legged Deadlift	Back	118	10–15	3
Seated Curl	Biceps	50	10–15	3
Standing One-Leg Calf Raise	Calves	164	10–15	3

» Rest 45–60 seconds between each set   » Perform this routine twice weekly

ROUTINE B (CHEST, SHOULDERS, AND TRICEPS)

Exercise	Muscles Worked	Page	Reps	Sets
Incline Bench Press	Chest	150	8–12	3
Decline Bench Press	Chest	149	8–12	3
Flat Bench Fly	Chest	141	8–12	3
Seated Shoulder Press	Shoulders	212	8–12	4
Bent-Over Raise	Shoulders	196	10–12	2
Lying Extension	Triceps	75	8–12	3
Basic Kickback	Triceps	68	10–15	3

» Rest 45–60 seconds between each set   » Perform this routine twice weekly

INTERMEDIATE WORKOUT #2
ROUTINE A (ABS AND LEGS)

Exercise	Muscles Worked	Page	Reps	Sets
Double Crunch	Abs	33	10–12	3
Cycle Crunch	Abs	34	10–12	3
Squat	Legs	183	10–15	3
Lunge	Legs	169	10–15	3
Split Squat	Legs	186	10–15	3
Reverse Lunge	Legs	173	10–15	3
Standing One-Leg Calf Raise	Calves	164	10–15	3

>> *Rest 45–60 seconds between each set*   >> *Perform this routine once a week*

ROUTINE B (BACK AND CHEST)

Exercise	Muscles Worked	Page	Reps	Sets
Deadlift	Back	116	6–8	4
Chest Press	Chest	148	6–8	4
Basic Two-Arm Row	Back	104	8–10	4
Decline Bench Press	Chest	149	8–10	4
Pullover	Back	124	8–10	3
Incline Bench Fly	Chest	143	8–10	3

>> *Rest 45–60 seconds between each set*   >> *Perform this routine once a week*

ROUTINE C (SHOULDERS, BICEPS, AND TRICEPS)

Exercise	Muscles Worked	Page	Reps	Sets
Standing Shoulder Press	Shoulders	213	6–10	4
Seated Side Raise	Shoulders	221	8–10	3
Standing Bent-Over Raise	Shoulders	197	10–12	3
Biceps Curl	Biceps	45	6–8	3
Incline Hammer Curl	Biceps	55	8–10	3
Basic Kickback	Triceps	68	8–10	3
Incline Lying Extension	Triceps	78	8–10	3
Wrist Curl	Forearms	101	10–15	1
Wrist Extension	Forearms	102	10–15	1

>> *Rest 45–60 seconds between each set*   >> *Perform this routine once a week*

INTERMEDIATE "PLUS" WORKOUT #2

Your experience also lets you do some of the more difficult, multi-muscle exercises in this book—especially the "Combine and Conquer" moves that are found at the end of most of the sections. Combining them into one full-body workout may feel like a return to using the Beginner programs—since you need to work out only two or three times a week—but *this* full-body plan is only for those looking for extreme results.

Exercise	Muscles Worked	Page	Reps	Sets
Straight-Leg Crunch	Abs	35	8–10	3
Cycle Crunch	Abs	33	8–10	3
Squat Jump	Entire lower body	194	8–10	3
Lunge Front Squat	Legs and biceps	180	8–10	3
Power Clean and Press	Legs, shoulders, triceps, chest, back, abdominals, and glutes	122	8–10	3
Fly Press	Chest	156	8–10	3
Three-Stage Lateral Raise	Front, side, and rear deltoids	203	10–12	3
Curl and Press	Shoulders and biceps	65	10–12	2
Press Pullover	Triceps	83	10–12	2
Walking Calf Raise	Legs, calves, and forearms	168	10–12	2

» Rest 45–60 seconds between each superset   » Perform this routine three times weekly

Index

Boldface page references indicate photographs.
Underscored references indicate boxed text.

Push curl, 67, **67**

Push press, 215, **215**

Pushup

basic, 157, **157**

Multiply Your Moves!

techniques, 160

step decline, 158, **158**

step incline, 159, **159**

R

Range of motion, 9, 10

Repetitions

mini-reps, 238

number of, 255–56

Reverse crunch, 32, **32**

Reverse curl

basic, 47, **47**

concentration, 53, **53**

incline, 55, **55**

kneeling, 49, **49**

preacher, 86, **86**

incline bench, 90, **90**

Swiss-ball, 88, **88**

prone, 59, **59**

seated, 51, **51**

Swiss-ball, 57, 57

variations, 62

wall, 61, **61**

Romanian deadlift, single-leg, 123,

123

Row

back

basic two-arm, 104, **104**

flat bench, 107, **107**

incline bench, 108, **108**

one-arm, 106, **106**

seated bent-over, 105, **105**

back extension curl, 112,

112

kickback, 74, **74**

single-leg, single-arm, 114,

114

single-leg row, 113, **113**

Swiss-ball lateral, 115, **115**

upright, 137, **137**

Row/raise, seated, 202, **202**

S

Safety, 9–10

Scissor-kick crunch, 41, **41**

Seated curl, 50, **50**

hammer, 51, **51**

reverse, 51, **51**

Seated good morning, 136, **136**

Selectorized adjustable dumbbells,

15–17

Shoulders, exercises for

bent-over raise

basic, 196, **196**

lying flat bench, 199, **199**